Lecture Notes on
History Taking and Examination

Lecture Notes on History Taking and Examination

Robert Turner
MD, FRCP
Clinical Reader in Medicine and
Honorary Consultant Physician
Nuffield Department of Clinical Medicine
John Radcliffe Hospital, Oxford

Roger Blackwood
MA, FRCP
Consultant Physician
Wexham Park Hospital, Slough,
and Honorary Consultant Physician at
Hammersmith Hospital, London

SECOND EDITION

OXFORD

Blackwell Scientific Publications

LONDON EDINBURGH BOSTON

MELBOURNE PARIS BERLIN VIENNA

© 1983, 1991 by
Blackwell Scientific Publications
Editorial Offices:
Osney Mead, Oxford OX2 0EL
25 John Street, London WC1N 2BL
23 Ainslie Place, Edinburgh EH3 6AJ
238 Main Street, Cambridge
  Massachusetts 02142, USA
54 University Street, Carlton
  Victoria 3053, Australia

Other Editorial Offices:
Librairie Arnette SA
2, rue Casimir-Delavigne
75006 Paris
France

Blackwell Wissenschafts-Verlag
Meinekestrasse 4
D-1000 Berlin 15
Germany

Blackwell MZV
Feldgasse 13
A-1238 Wien
Austria

First published 1983
Second edition 1991
Reprinted 1992, 1993
Four Dragons edition 1991
Reprinted 1993

Set by Times Graphics, Singapore
Printed and bound in Great Britain at
The Alden Press, Oxford

DISTRIBUTORS

  Marston Book Services Ltd
  PO Box 87
  Oxford OX2 0DT
  (*Orders*: Tel: 0865 791155
          Fax: 0865 791927
          Telex: 837515)

USA
  Blackwell Scientific Publications, Inc.
  238 Main Street
  Cambridge, MA 02142
  (*Orders*: Tel: 800 759-6102
          617 876-7000)

Canada
  Times Mirror Professional Publishing, Ltd
  130 Flaska Drive
  Markham, Ontario L6G 1B8
  (*Orders*: Tel: 800 268-4178
          416 470-6739)

Australia
  Blackwell Scientific Publications Pty Ltd
  54 University Street
  Carlton, Victoria 3053
  (*Orders*: Tel: 03 347-5552)

British Library
Cataloguing in Publication Data

Turner, Robert, *1938–*
  Lecture notes on history taking and
  examination.—2nd ed.
  1. Medicine. Physical examination.
  Techniques
  I. Title II. Blackwood, Roger, *1945–*
  616.0754

  ISBN 0-632-02854-8 (BSP)
       0-632-02885-8 (Four Dragons)

Contents

Preface, vii

Introduction; The First Approach, 1

1 History Taking, 4

2 General Examination, 19

3 Examination of the Cardiovascular System, 33

4 Examination of the Chest, 55

5 Examination of the Abdomen, 65

6 Examination of the Nervous System, 76

7 Basic Examination, Notes and Diagnostic Principles, 108

8 Assessment of Disability Including Care of the Elderly, 118

9 Communicating, 124

10 Clinical Investigations, 130

11 The 12-Lead Electrocardiogram, 159

12 The Interpretation of Investigations, 185

13 Laboratory Results — Normal Values, 187

Index, 193

Preface

When a medical student first approaches a patient, he has to develop a suitable doctor–patient relationship, master many relevant skills and techniques, and develop an enquiring and intelligent approach. These notes are intended to assist with all these aspects, but particularly they aim to inform the student succinctly of what he should do, and how he should think, at each stage.

It is intended that the book be easily pocketed, and that it could be read near to the bedside. In general the pages are arranged with simple instructions on the left, with important aspects requiring action marked with a dot (•). On the right are brief details of clinical situations and diseases which are relevant to abnormal findings. Subsidiary lists are marked with a dash (—). Although the notes could be simply used as a manual, it is hoped that the student will quickly learn the art of altering his approach appropriately, according to the specific manifestations of illness and the personality of the patient.

The notes have been used in the Oxford Clinical Medical School for 14 years. We much appreciate the invaluable guidance and comments we have received from many colleagues and students. Different doctors use slightly different techniques in taking a history and examination, and inevitably some would prefer slightly different instructions.

Throughout the text the pronoun he is used to refer to doctors, students and patients. This is not intended to imply that all doctors, students and patients are male and we hope the reader is not offended by what has been adopted as an economical linguistic convention.

Robert Turner
Roger Blackwood
Oxford 1990

Introduction
The First Approach

GENERAL PRINCIPLES

When the student (or doctor) approaches a patient there are *three initial objectives:*
- Obtain professional rapport with patient and gain his confidence.
- Obtain all relevant information which allow assessment of his illness, and provisional diagnoses.
- Obtain general information regarding the patient, his background, social situation and problems. In particular it is necessary to find out how the illness has affected him and his life. The assessment of the patient as a whole is of utmost importance.

The following notes provide a guide as to how one obtains the necessary information. *In taking a history or making an examination there are two complementary aims:*
- Obtain all possible information about a patient and his illness (a 'data base').
- Solve the problem as to the diagnoses.

For each symptom or sign one needs to think of a differential diagnosis, and of other relevant information (by history, examination or investigation) which one will need to support or to refute these possible diagnoses. A good history combines these two facets, and one should never approach the patient with just a set series of rote questions. However, until one knows more medicine, one cannot know the possible significance of the information one gains, and the obvious change of questioning which this might entail. These notes provide background information enabling a full history and examination to be taken. This provides a necessary basis for a later, more inquisitive approach which should develop as knowledge about illnesses is acquired.

The student must take his own history, make his own examination and write his own clinical records. After 1 month he should be sufficiently proficient that his notes could become the final hospital record. The student should add a summary including his assessment of the problem list, provisional diagnoses and preliminary investigations. Initially these will be incomplete and occasionally incorrect. Nevertheless, this exercise will help to inculcate an enquiring approach and to high-light areas in which further questioning, investigation or reading is needed.

Training to become a doctor includes the distinct challenges of learning:

— to have a natural, sincere, receptive and when necessary supportive relationship with patients and staff;
— to obtain wide experience of clinical diseases, how they affect patients and how they are managed;
— the optimum means of working with patients and colleagues to facilitate good care;
— to understand the scientific background of disease including the advances which are being made and how these can be applied to improve care.

Your clinical skills and knowledge can develop with good organisation.

• *Take advantage of seeing many patients* in hospital, in clinics and in the community. It is particularly helpful to be present when patients are being admitted with emergencies or are being seen in a clinic for the first time.

Medicine is a practical subject and first-hand experience is invaluable. The more patients you can clerk yourself, the sooner you will become proficient and the more you will learn about patients and their diseases.

• *Choose a medium-size student's text book* in which you read up about each disease you see or each problem which you encounter.

Attaching knowledge to individual patients is a great help in acquiring and remembering facts. 'To practise medicine without a text book is like a sailor without a chart, whereas to study books rather than patients is like a sailor who does not go to sea.'

• *Regularly pick up and read the editorials* or any articles which interest you in a general medical journal such as *New England Journal of Medicine, Lancet* or *British Medical Journal*.

Even if at first you are not able to put information into context, they will keep you in touch with new developments that add interest. Nevertheless, it is not sensible to delve too deeply into any one subject when you are just beginning.

At first medicine seems a huge subject and each fact you learn seems to be an isolated piece of information. How will you ever be able to learn what is required? You will find after a few months that the bits of information do inter-relate and that you are able to put new bits of information into context. The pieces of the jig-saw puzzle begin to fit together and then your confidence will increase. Although you will need to learn many facts, equally important is to acquire the attitude of questioning, reasoning and knowing when and where to go to seek additional information.

At the basis of all medicine is clinical competence. No amount of knowledge will make up for poor clinical technique. Over the first few weeks it is essential to learn the 'ABC' of clinical medicine, covered in these notes.

— How to relate to patients.
— How to take a good history efficiently, knowing which question to ask next and to avoid asking leading questions.
— How to examine patients in a logical manner, in a set routine which will mean you will not miss an unexpected sign.

You will be surprised how often students can fail an exam, not because of lack of knowledge but because they have not mastered elementary clinical skills. These notes are written to try to help you to identify what is important and to help to relate findings to common clinical situations. There is nothing inherently difficult about clinical medicine. You will quickly become clinically competent if you apply yourself, including initially learning by rote which skills are appropriate for each situation and using the available clinical opportunities.

A later chapter covers aspects of presentation of your findings and communication. Brief introductory information about several common clinical tests is given, together with a simple guide to reading an electrocardiogram (ECG). In the meantime, we wish you 'good luck' with your career and acquiring the basic clinical skills.

Chapter 1
History Taking

GENERAL COMMENTS

- Look the part of a doctor and put the patient at ease. Be confident and quietly friendly.
- Greet the patient 'Good morning, Mr Smith'.
- Shake the patient's hand or place your hand on his if he is ill.
- State your name and that you are a student doctor helping staff care for patients.
- Make sure the patient is comfortable.
- Explain that you wish to ask the patient questions to find out what happened to him.
- Let the patient tell his story in his own words as much as possible. At first listen and then take discreet notes as he talks.
- Try to conduct a conversation rather than an interrogation, following the patient's trains of thought as much as possible.
- Beware pseudomedical terms, e.g. 'gastric flu'.
- Do not ask leading questions.

    Leading questions can produce incorrect or misleading answers. Open-ended questions or questions suggesting an answer opposite to that expected are better, e.g. do not ask a thyrotoxic patient 'Do you find hot weather uncomfortable?' but either 'Do you dislike hot or cold weather?' or 'Do you like hot weather?'

    Patients are variable witnesses; some are reluctant, some emotional, some irrelevant in their history. Different approaches are therefore needed in different circumstances. You must be sensitive to a patient's mood and non-verbal responses, e.g. hesitancy revealing emotional content. Be understanding, receptive and matter of fact without excessive overt sympathy. Rarely show surprise or reproach.

Usual sequence of events

History	***The history is of prime importance:***
↓	— what has happened
Examination	— what kind of person
↓	— how the illness has affected him and his
Problem list	family
↓	— his physical and social environment
Differential	— establishes physician/patient relationship
diagnosis	— *often gives diagnosis.*
↓	
Investigations	
↓	
Diagnosis confirmed	
↓	
Treatment	

Usual sequence of history
- Nature of principal complaints, e.g. chest pain, poor home circumstances.
- History of present complaint — details of current illness.
- Enquiry of other symptoms (see Functional enquiry, p. 7).
- Past history.
- Family history.
- Personal and social history.

If one's initial enquiries make it apparent that one section is of more importance than usual (e.g. previous relevant illnesses or operation), then relevant enquiries can be brought forward to an earlier stage in the history (e.g. past history after finding principal complaints).

Find principal symptoms
- *Find the principal symptoms or symptom* by asking:
  - 'Of what do you complain?' *or*
  - 'What made you go to the doctor?'
     Do not say:
     'What's wrong?' *or*
     'What brought you here?'

- **Start your written history with a single sentence** summing up what your patient is complaining of. It should be like the banner headline of a newspaper. For example:

c/o chest pain for 6 months.

History of present illness

- **Determine the chronology of the illness** by asking:
  - 'How and when did your illness begin' *or*
  - 'When did you first notice anything wrong?' *or*
  - 'When did you last feel completely well?'
- **Begin by stating when the patient was last perfectly well.** Symptoms should then be described in **chronological order of onset.** Both the *date of onset* and the *length of time* prior to admission should be recorded. Symptoms should never be dated by the day of the week as this later becomes meaningless.
- **Obtain a detailed description of each symptom** by asking:
  - e.g. 'Tell me what the pain was like'. Make sure you ask about all symptoms whether they seem relevant or not.
- **With all symptoms obtain the following details.**
  - Duration.
  - Onset — sudden or gradual.
  - What has happened since — constant or periodic
    - frequency
    - getting worse or better.
  - Precipitating or relieving factors.
  - Associated symptoms.
- **If pain is a symptom also determine the following.**
  - Site.
  - Radiation.
  - Character, e.g. ache, pressure, shooting, stabbing, dull.
  - Severity, e.g. 'Did it interfere with what you were doing? Does it keep you awake?'

    Avoid technical language when describing a patient's history. Do not say 'the patient complained of melaena' rather 'the patient complained of passing loose, black, tarry motions'.

    When patients are unable to give an adequate or reliable history, the necessary information must be obtained from friends or relations. Accordingly, the student should arrange with the houseman to be present when the relatives are interviewed. This is particularly important with patients suffering from disease of the central nervous system. The source of such information should be stated.

FUNCTIONAL ENQUIRY

This is a check list of symptoms not already discovered. Do not ask questions already covered in establishing the principal symptoms. This list may detect other symptoms. Modify your questioning according to the nature of the suspected disease, time available and circumstances. If during the functional enquiry a positive answer is obtained, full details must be elicited. The stars (*) denote questions which must nearly always be asked.

General questions
- Ask about the following symptoms.
  - * Appetite: 'What is your appetite like? Do you feel like eating?'
  - * Weight: 'Have you lost or gained weight recently?'
  - * General wellbeing: 'Do you feel well in yourself?'
  - Fatigue: 'Are you more or less tired than you used to be?'
  - Fever or chills: 'Have you felt hot or cold? Have you shivered?'
  - Night sweats: 'Have you noticed any sweating at night or any other time?'
  - Aches or pains.
  - Rash: 'Have you had any rash recently? Does it itch?'
  - Lumps and bumps.

Cardiovascular and respiratory system
- Ask about the following symptoms.
  - * Chest pain: 'Have you any recent pains or discomfort in the chest?'

    The most common causes of chest pain are:

    Ischaemic heart disease: severe constricting, central chest pain radiating to neck, jaw and left arm. *Angina* is this pain precipitated by exercise or emotion; relieved by rest. In a *myocardial infarction* the pain may come on at rest, be more severe, and last hours.

Pleuritic pain: sharp, localised pain, usually lateral; worse on inspiration or cough.

— * Short of breath: 'Are you breathless at any time?'

Breathlessness (*dyspnoea*) and chest pain must be accurately described and the *degree of exercise* which brings on the symptoms must be noted (e.g. climbing one flight of stairs, after ¼-mile walk).

— Short of breath on lying flat — *orthopnoea*: 'Do you get breathless in bed? What do you do then? Does it get worse or better on sitting up? How many pillows do you use? Can you sleep without them?'

— Waking up breathless — *paroxysmal nocturnal dyspnoea*: 'Do you wake at night with any symptoms? Do you gasp for breath? What do you do then?'

Orthopnoea (breathless when lying flat) and paroxysmal nocturnal dyspnoea (waking up breathless, relieved on sitting up) are features of *left heart failure*.

— * Ankle swelling.

Common in *congestive cardiac failure* (right heart failure).

— Palpitations: 'Are you aware of your heart beating?'

Palpitations may be — single thumps (*ectopics?*)

— slow or fast

— regular or irregular.

Ask patient to tap them out.

Paroxysmal tachycardia (sudden attacks of palpitations) usually starts and finishes abruptly.

— * Cough: 'Do you have a cough? Is it a dry cough or do you cough up sputum? When do you cough?'

— Sputum: 'What colour is your sputum? How much do you cough up?'

Green sputum usually indicates an *acute chest infection*. Clear sputum daily during winter months suggests *chronic bronchitis*. Frothy sputum suggests *left heart failure*.

— * Blood in sputum — haemoptysis: 'Have you coughed up blood?'

Haemoptysis must be taken very seriously. Causes include:

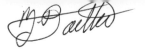

> — *carcinoma of bronchus*
> — *pulmonary embolism*
> — *mitral stenosis*
> — *tuberculosis*
> — *bronchiectasis.*

— Blackouts — *syncope*: 'Have you had any blackouts or faints? Did you feel light-headed or did the room go round? Did you lose consciousness? Did you have warning? Can you remember what happened?'
— * Smoking: 'Do you smoke? How many cigarettes do you smoke?'

Gastrointestinal system

- Ask about the following points.
   — Nausea: 'Are there times when you feel sick?'
   — Vomiting: 'Do you vomit? What is it like?'

> *'Coffee grounds' vomit* suggests altered blood. If old food is seen, *pyloric stenosis* is present. If blood has been vomited, what colour is it — dark or bright red?

   — Difficulty in swallowing — *dysphagia*: 'Do you have difficulty swallowing? Where does it stick?'

> For solids: often organic obstruction.
> For fluids: often neurological or psychological.

   — Indigestion: 'Do you have any discomfort in your stomach after eating?'
   — Abdominal pain: 'Where is the pain? What is its relation to meals or opening your bowels? What relieves the pain?'
   — * Bowel habit: 'Are your bowels all right?'

> If *diarrhoea* is suggested, the number of motions per day and their nature (blood? pus? mucous?) must be established. 'What are your motions like' The stools may be pale, bulky and float (fat in stool — *steatorrhoea*) or tarry from digested blood (*melaena* —usually from upper gastrointestinal tract). Bright blood on the surface of a motion may be from *haemorrhoids*, whereas blood in a stool may signify *cancer* or *inflammatory bowel disease.*

   — Jaundice: 'Is your urine dark? Are your stools pale? What tablets have you been taking recently? Have you have any recent injections or transfusions? Have you been abroad recently? How much alcohol do you drink?'

Jaundice may be:

Obstructive (dark urine pale stools) from:

— *carcinoma* of the *head* of the *pancreas*

— *gallstones.*

Heptocellular (dark urine, pale stools may develop) from:

— ethanol (*cirrhosis*)

— drugs or transfusions (*serum hepatitis)*

— drug reactions or infections (travel abroad, *viral hepatitis* or *amoebae).*

Haemolytic jaundice

— unconjugated bilirubin is bound to albumin and is not secreted in the urine (*acholuric jaundice).*

Genito-urinary system

- Ask about the following points.

— Loin pain: 'Any pain in your back?'

  Pain in the loins suggests pyelonephritis.

— * Urine: 'Are your waterworks alright? Do you pass a lot of water at night? Do you have any difficulty passing water? Is there blood in your water?'

  Polyuria and *nocturia* occur in *diabetes. Prostatism* results in slow onset of urination, a poor stream and terminal dribbling.

— Sex: 'Any problem with sex?'

— * Menstruation: 'Any problems with your periods? Do you bleed heavily? Do you bleed between periods?'

  Vaginal bleeding between periods or after the menopause raises the possibility of *cervical* or *uterine cancer.*

— Vaginal discharge.

— Pain on intercourse (*dyspareunia).*

Nervous system

- Ask about the following points.

— * Headache: 'Do you have any headaches? Where are they?'

  Headaches are often *tension* in origin and either frontal or occipital. Occipital headache on waking may be due to *raised intracranial pressure* (e.g. from a *tumour* or *malignant hypertension*).

— Vision: 'Do you have any blurred or double vision?'
— Hearing.
— Dizziness: 'Do you have any dizziness or episodes when the world goes round (*vertigo*)?'

> Dizziness with light-headed symptoms, when sudden in onset, may be cardiac (enquire about palpitations). When slow onset may be vasovagal 'fainting' or an internal haemorrhage or bleed.
>
> Vertigo may be from *ear disease* (enquire about deafness earache or discharge) or *brainstem dysfunction*.

— Unsteady gait: 'Any difficulty walking or running?'
— Weakness.
— Numbness or increased sensation: 'Any patches of numbness?'
— Pins and needles.
— Sphincter disturbance: 'Any difficulties holding your water/bowels?'
— * Depression: 'How is your mood? Happy or unhappy? If depressed, how much? How do you feel about the future? Is this how you often feel? What is duration? What do you think is the cause? How long have you felt like this?'

> Enquire interest, concentration, irritability, feelings of guilt.

— * Worry and anxiety: 'Do you tend to worry? Are there times when you feel anxious or tense? Any worries in your job or family? Any financial worries?'
— Sleep: 'Any difficulties sleeping? Do you have difficulty getting to sleep? Do you wake early?'

> Difficulties of sleep are commonly associated with depression or anxiety.

— Fits or faints: 'Have you had any funny episodes?'

The following details should be sought from the patient and any observer — duration

> — frequency and length of attacks
> — time of attacks, e.g. if standing, at night
> — mode of onset and termination
> — premonition or aura, light-headed or vertigo
> — biting of tongue, loss of sphincter control, injury, etc.

Grand mal epilepsy classically produces sudden unconsciousness without any warning and on waking the patient
feels drowsy with a headache, sore tongue, and has been
incontinent.

Locomotor system

• Ask about pain, stiffness, or swelling of joints: 'When and how did it
start?' 'Have you injured the joint?'

There are innumerable causes of *arthritis* (painful, swollen,
tender joints) and *arthralgia* (painful joints). Patients may
incorrectly attribute a problem to some injury.

Osteoarthritis is a joint 'wearing out', and is often
asymmetric involving weight-bearing joints such as hip or
knee. Exercise makes the joint pain worse.

Rheumatoid arthritis is a generalised 'autoimmune disease' with symmetrical involvement. In the hands, fusiform
swelling of the interphalangeal joints is accompanied by
swollen metacarpophalangeal joints. Large joints are often
affected. Stiffness is worse after rest, e.g. on waking and
improves with use.

Gout usually involves a single joint, such as the first
metatarsal-phalangeal joint, but can lead to gross hand
involvement with asymmetric uric acid lumps (*tophi*) by
some joints, and in the tips of the ears.

• Assess functional disability: 'How far can you walk? Can you walk
upstairs? Is any particular movement difficult? Can you dress yourself?
How long does it take?'

Thyroid disease

• Ask about the following points.
  — Weight change.
  — Reaction to the weather: 'Do you dislike the hot or cold weather?'
  — Irritability: 'Are you more or less irritable compared with a few
    years ago?'
  — Diarrhoea/constipation.
  — Palpitations.
  — Dry skin or greasy hair: 'Is your skin dry or greasy? Is your hair
    dry or greasy?'

— Depression.
— Croaky voice.

> *Hypothyroid patients* put on weight without increase in appetite, dislike cold weather, have dry skin and thin, dry hair, a puffy face, a croaky voice, are usually calm and may be depressed.
>
> *Hyperthyroid patients* may lose weight despite eating more, dislike hot weather, perspire excessively, have palpitations, a tremor, may be agitated and tearful. Young people have predominantly nervous and heat intolerance symptoms, whereas old people tend to present with cardiac symptoms.

PAST HISTORY

The past history should include an account of all previous illnesses or operations, whether apparently important or not. For instance, a casually mentioned attack of influenza or chill may have been a manifestation of an occult infection. Some idea of the importance of a past illness may be gained by finding out how long the patient was in bed or off work. Complications of any previous illnesses should be carefully enquired into and, here, leading questions are some times necessary.

General questions

• Ask about the following.
  — 'Have you had any serious illnesses in your life?''
  — 'Have you had any emotional or nervous problems?'
  — 'Have you had any operations?
  — 'Have you ever had — *rheumatic fever?*
    — *kidney problems?*
    — *jaundice?*
    — *TB?*
    — *tropical illnesses?*
    — *allergies, e.g. hayfever?'*

The latter questions may not always be relevant; e.g. if the problem seems to be *high blood pressure* it is important to ask about kidney problems.

If the patient's history suggests cardiac failure, you must ask if he has had *rheumatic fever*.

Patients have often had examinations for life insurance or the armed forces.

— 'Have any medicines ever upset you?'

Allergic responses to drugs may include an itchy rash, vomiting, diarrhoea, or severe illness including jaundice. Many patients claim to be allergic but are not. An accurate description of the supposed allergic episodes is important.

FAMILY HISTORY

Family history gives clues to possible predisposition to illness (e.g. heart attacks) *and whether a patient may have reason to be particularly anxious about a certain disease*, (e.g. mother died of cancer). Death certificates and patient knowledge are often inaccurate. Patients may be reluctant to talk about relatives' illnesses if they were mental diseases, epilepsy or cancer.

General questions

- Ask about the following.
  - 'Are your parents alive? Are they fit and well? What did your parents die from?'
  - 'Have you any brothers or sisters? Are they fit and well?'
  - Do you have any children? Are they fit and well?'
  - Is there any history of — heart trouble?

                                   — diabetes?

                                   — blood pressure in the family?'

This latter question can be varied to take account of the patient's major complaint.

PERSONAL AND SOCIAL HISTORY

One needs to find out what kind of person the patient is, what his home circumstances are and how his illness has affected him and his family. Your aim is to understand the patient's illness in the context of his personality and his home environment. You want to know if he can convalesce satisfactorily at home and at what stage. What are the consequences of his illness? Will advice, information and help be needed? An interview with a relative or friend may be very helpful.

General questions
- Ask about the following.
  - Family: 'Is everything alright at home? Do you have any family problems?'

    It may be appropriate to ask 'What is your marriage like? Is sex all right?' Problems may arise from physical or emotional reasons, and the patient may appreciate an opportunity to discuss worries.
  - Accommodation: 'Where do you live?' 'Is it all right?'
  - Job: 'What is your job? Could you tell me exactly what you do? Is it satisfactory?' Will your illness affect your work?'
  - Hobbies: 'What do you do in your spare time? Do you have any social life?'
  - Alcohol: 'How much alcohol do you drink?'

    Alcoholics usually underestimate their daily consumption. It may be helpful to go through a 'drinking day'. If there is a suspicion of a drinking problem, you can ask 'Do you ever drink in the morning? Do you worry about controlling your drinking? Does it affect your job, home or social life?'
  - Smoking: 'Do you smoke?' Have you ever smoked? Why did you give up? How many cigarettes do you smoke a day?'

    Particularly relevant for heart or chest disease but must always be asked.
  - Drugs: 'What pills are you taking at the moment? Have you taken any other pills in the last few months?'

    This is an extremely important question. A complete list of all drugs and doses must be obtained.

    If relevant ask about any pets, visits abroad, previous or present exposure during working to coaldust, asbestos, etc.

Having taken the history, you should have some idea of possible diagnoses, and an assessment of the patient as a person. You will know which systems you wish to concentrate on when examining the patient. Further relevant questions to ask the patient may arise from abnormalities found on examination or investigation.

Either now or after examining the patient it can be helpful to ask:
- 'What do you think is wrong with you?'
- 'Have you any questions?'

A specimen history is given below.

SPECIMEN HISTORY

Mr John Smith.
Aged 52. Machine operator. Oxford.
c/o severe chest pain for 2 hours.

History of present illness (HPI)

The patient was perfectly well until 6 months ago. He then began to notice central, dull chest ache, occasionally felt in the jaw, coming on when walking about ½ mile, worse when going uphill and worse in cold weather. When he stopped the pain went off after 2 minutes. The patient found glyceryl trinitrate tablets (GTN) relieved the pain rapidly. In the last month the pain came on with less exercise after 100 yards.

Today at 10 am whilst sitting at work the chest pain came on without provocation. It was the worst pain he had ever experienced in his life and he thought he was going to die. The pain was central, crushing in nature, radiating to the left arm and neck and with it the feeling of nausea and sweating. The patient was rushed to hospital where he received an intravenous injection of diamorphine which rapidly relieved the pain. An electrocardiogram confirmed a myocardial infarction and the patient was admitted to the coronary care unit.

The patient had noticed very mild breathlessness on exertion for 3 months, but had not experienced palpitations, dizziness, breathlessness on lying flat, ankle swelling or coughing. On one occasion, however, 2 weeks ago the patient had woken with a suffocating feeling and had

had to sit on the edge of the bed and subsequently open the bedroom window in order to get his breath. This had not recurred and he did not report it to his doctor.

Functional enquiry
RS (respiratory system)

> Morning cough over the last 3–4 winters with production of a small amount of clear sputum.
>
> No haemoptysis.

GI (gastrointestinal)

> Occasional mild indigestion.
>
> Bowels regular.
>
> Appetite normal.
>
> No other abnormalities.

GU (genito-urinary)

> No difficulties with micturition.
>
> Normal sex life.

NS (nervous system)

> Infrequent frontal headaches at the end of a hectic day. Otherwise no abnormalities

Past medical history
Fifteen years ago, appendicectomy. No complications.
No other operations or serious illnesses.
No history of rheumatic fever, nephritis or hypertension.
Never been abroad.

Family history
Father died aged 73 — 'heart attack'.
Mother died aged 71 — 'cancer'.
Two brothers fit and well (aged 48 and 46).
Two sons (aged 23, 25) both fit and well.
No family history of diabetes or hypertension.

Personal and social history
Happy both at work and home. Both sons married and living in Oxford. Wife works as an office cleaner. No financial difficulties.

Smokes 20 cigarettes per day. Two pints of beer on Saturdays only.

Patient always worked as machine operator since leaving school except for 2 years National Service spent entirely in the UK.

Medication

Other than glyceryl trinitrate, no drugs currently being taken.

Chapter 2
General Examination

The initial assessment of the patient will have been made whilst taking a history. The general appearance of the patient is the first observation, and thereafter the order of examination will vary. The system to which the presenting symptoms refer is often examined first. Otherwise devise your own routine, examining each part of the body in turn, covering all systems. An example is:

- — general appearance
- — hands and nails
- — radial pulse
- — axillary nodes
- — cervical lymph nodes
- — facies — conjunctivae — tongue
- — jugular venous pressure
- — heart — breasts
- — respiratory system
- — spine (whilst patient sitting forward)
- — abdomen including femoral pulses
- — legs
- — nervous system
- — rectal or pelvic examination
- — gait.

Whichever part of the body one is examining, one should always use the same routine.
1 *Inspection.*
2 *Palpation.*
3 *Percussion.*
4 *Auscultation.*

GENERAL INSPECTION

The beginning of the examination is a careful observation of the patient as a whole.

Note the following.

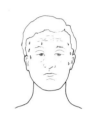

- *Does the patient look ill?*
  - what age does he look?
  - febrile, hydrated
  - alert, confused, drowsy, resentful
  - intelligent, co-operative, happy, sad
  - fat, muscular, or wasted.
- *Skin:*
  - colour
  - texture.
- *Rash* — if so, what is it like? Describe:
  - position
  - size of lesions
  - discrete or confluent
  - flat, impalpable—macular
  - raised — papular: in skin, localised
    - plaque: larger, e.g. >0.5 cm
    - nodules: deeper in dermis
    - wheal: oedema fluid
    - vesicles: contain fluid
    - bullae: large vesicles, e.g. >0.5 cm
    - pustular.
  - is edge well demarcated?
  - colour
  - surface, e.g. scaling, shiny
  - temperature
  - tender
  - blanches on pressure: *petechiae* are small, red haemorrhages, non-tender macules, which do not blanche on pressure.

HANDS

Note the following.
- *Temperature:*
  - unduly cold hands — *?low cardiac output*
  - unduly warm hands — *?high output state,* e.g. thyrotoxicosis
  - cold and sweaty   — *anxiety* or other causes of *sympathetic overactivity,* e.g. hypoglycaemia.
- *Nails:*
  - bitten
  - leuconychia — white nails
    - can occur in *cirrhosis*
  - koilonychia — misshapen, concave nails
    - can occur in *iron deficiency anaemia*

Normal

Koilonychia

  - clubbing   — loss of angle at base of nail
    - occurs in specific diseases:

Clubbing

Heart: *infectious endocarditis; cyanotic congenital heart disease.*
Lungs: *carcinoma of the bronchus* (chronic infection — *abscess; bronchiectasis,* e.g. *cystic fibrosis; empyema); fibrosing alveolitis* (not chronic bronchitis).
Liver: *cirrhosis.*
Crohn's disease.
Congenital.
  - splinter haemorrhages — occur in *infectious endocarditis* but are more common in people doing manual work.

Splinter haemorrhages

  - Osler's nodes — red painful lumps in finger pulp in *infectious endocarditis.*

- *Palms:*
  - erythema — can be normal, also occurs with *chronic liver disease, pregnancy.*

  - Dupuytren's contracture — tethering of skin in palm to flexor tendon of fourth finger.
    - can occur in *cirrhosis.*
- *Joints:*
  - symmetrical swellings occur in *rheumatoid arthritis*
  - asymmetrical swellings occur in *gout* and *osteoarthritis.*

MOUTH

Look at the following.
- *Tongue:*
  - cyanosed, moist.

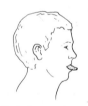

Central cyanosis

Cyanosis is a reduction in the oxygenation of the blood, with more than 5 g/dl deoxygenated haemoglobin.

Central cyanosis (blue tongue) denotes a right-to-left shunt (unsaturated blood appearing in systemic circulation):
- congenital heart disease, e.g. *Fallot's tetralogy*
- lung disease, e.g. *obstructive airways disease.*

Peripheral cyanosis (blue fingers, pink tongue) denotes inadequate peripheral circulation.

A dry tongue can mean salt and water deficiency (often called 'dehydration') but also occurs with mouth breathing.

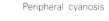

Peripheral cyanosis

- *Teeth:*
  - natural, false, rotten.

- *Gums:*
  — bleeding, swollen.
- *Throat:*
  — tonsils, sore throat.
- *Smell his breath:*
  — ketosis
  — alcohol
  — foetor — constipation, appendicitis
          — musty in liver failure.

> *Ketosis* is a sweet-smelling breath occurring with *starvation* or *severe diabetes*.
>
> *Hepatic foetor* is a musty smell in *liver failure*.

EYES

- Look at the eyes:
  — sclera — icterus
  — lower lid conjunctiva — anaemia

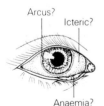

Arcus?
Icteric?
Anaemia?

> The most obvious demonstration of *jaundice* is the yellow colour of the conjunctivae (*icteric*). *Anaemia*. If the lower lid is everted, the colour of the mucous membrane can easily be seen. If these are pale the haemoglobin is usually less than 9 g %.
>
> An *arcus senilis* is a white line round the cornea which, although common and of little significance in the elderly, suggests *hyperlipidaemia* in younger patients.
>
> *Hypercalcaemia* may give a vertical line in exposed part of cornea.

EXAMINE FOR PALPABLE LYMPH NODES

- In the neck:
  — above clavicle (posterior triangle)

— medial to sternomastoid area (anterior triangle)
— submandibular (can palpate submandibular gland)
— occipital.

These glands are best felt by sitting the patient up and examining from behind.

Left supraclavicular node can occur from spread of gastrointestinal malignancy (*Virchow's node*).

- In *axillae:*
  — abduct arm, insert your hand along lateral side of axilla, and

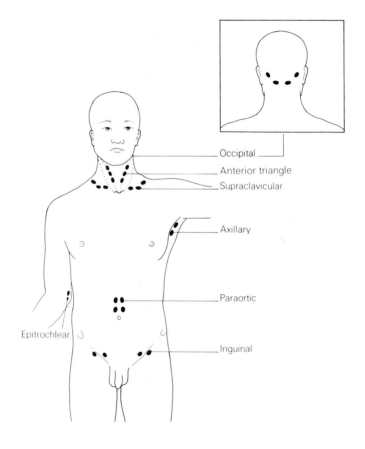

Occipital

Anterior triangle

Supraclavicular

Axillary

Paraortic

Epitrochlear

Inguinal

adduct arm, thus placing your finger-tips in the apex of the axilla. Palpate gently.
- In the *epitrochlear region:*
  - medial to and above elbow.
- In *groins:*
  - over inguinal ligament.
- In the *abdomen:*
  - usually very difficult to feel; some claim to have felt para-aortic nodes.

    Axillae often have soft, fleshy lymph nodes.

    Groins often have small, shotty nodes.

    Generalised large, rubbery nodes suggest *lymphoma.*

    Localised hard nodes suggest *cancer.*

    Tender nodes suggest *infection.*

    If many nodes are palpable — examine spleen and look for anaemia. *Reticulosis* or *leukaemia?*

LUMPS

- If there is an unusual lump, note:
  - site
  - size — measure in centimetres
  - shape, including nature of surface
  - fixed or mobile
  - consistency, e.g. cystic or solid, soft or hard, fluctuance
  - tender
  - pulsatile
  - transillumination.

    A *cancer* is usually hard, non-tender, irregular, fixed to neighbouring tissues, and possibly ulcerating skin.

    A *cyst* may have: — fluctuance: pressure across cyst will cause it to bulge in another plane.
    — transillumination: a light can be seen through it (usually only if room is darkened).
- Look at neighbouring lymph nodes. May find:
  - spread from cancer
  - inflamed lymph nodes from infection

BREASTS

Routinely the female breasts can be *briefly* inspected and palpated before or after examining the praecordium.
- Brief inspection for asymmetry, obvious lumps or inverted nipples. Occasionally skin changes may be seen.
- Palpate each half of both breasts with the flat of hand (fingers together, nearly extended with gentle pressure exerted from metacarpophalangeal joints) avoiding excessive pressure on the nipple. Note tenderness of lumps.

If the patient has a symptom, or a lump is found, then do a *full examination*.
- *Inspect:*
  - sitting up and ask to raise hands
  - differing size or shape
  - rashes, redness (abscess).
      Breast cancer — skin tethering
                    — peau d'orange (oedema of skin)
                    — nipple deviated or inverted.
- *Palpation:*
  - patient lying flat, one pillow
  - examine each breast with flat of hand, each quadrant in turn.
  If abnormal lump:
  - examine as for any lump (see above), bimanually if large. Is lump attached to skin or muscles?
  - lymph nodes — axilla
                — supraclavicular.
  - feel liver.

THYROID

- Inspect: then ask the patient to swallow, having given him a glass of water. Is there a lump? Does it move upwards on swallowing?
- Palpate bimanually: stand behind the patient and palpate with fingers

of both hands. Is the thyroid of normal size, shape and texture?
   If one lump is felt:
- Is thyroid multinodular?
- Does lump feel cystic?
- Ask patient to swallow — does thyroid rise normally?
- Is thyroid fixed?
- Can you get below the lump? If not, percuss over upper sternum for retrosternal extension.
- Are there cervical lymph nodes?

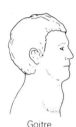
Goitre

The thyroid is normally soft. If there is a goitre (swelling of thyroid) assess if the swelling is:
— localised, e.g. *thyroid cyst*, *adenoma* or *carcinoma*
— generalised, e.g. *autoimmune thyroiditis*, *thyrotoxicosis*
— multinodular.
A swelling does not mean the gland is under- or over-active. In many cases the patient may be euthyroid.
The thyroid becomes slightly enlarged in pregnancy.

- If possibility of *thyrotoxic*, look for:
  — warm hands
  — perspiration
  — tremor
  — tachycardia, sinus rhythm or atrial fibrillation
  — wide, palpebral fissure or lid lag
  — thyroid bruit (on auscultation).

  Endocrine exophthalmos (may be associated with thyrotoxicosis):
  — conjunctival oedema: chemosis
  — proptosis: eye pushed forwards
  — deficient upward gaze and convergence
  — diplopia
  — papilloedema.

- If possibility of *hypothyroid*, look for:
  - dry hair and skin
  - xanthelasma
  - puffy face
  - croaky voice
  - delayed relaxation of supinator or ankle jerks.

OTHER ENDOCRINE DISEASES

Acromegaly
  - Enlarged soft tissue of hands, feet, face.
  - Coarse features, thick, greasy skin, large tongue (and other organs, e.g. thyroid).
  - Bitemporal hemianopia (from tumour pressing on optic chiasma).

Hypopituitary
  - No skin pigmentation.
  - Thin skin.
  - Decreased secondary sexual hair or delayed puberty.
  - Short stature (and on X-ray delayed fusion of epiphyses).
  - Bitemporal hemianopia if pituitary tumour.

Addison's disease
  - Increase skin pigmentation, including non-exposed areas, e.g. buccal pigmentation.
  - Postural hypotension.
  - If female, decreased body hair.

Cushing's syndrome
  - Truncal obesity, round, red face with hirsutes.
  - Thin skin and bruising, pink striae, hypertension.
  - Proximal muscle weakness.

Diabetes
Diabetic complications include:
  - Skin lesions — necrobiosis lipoidica.

— Ischaemic legs — diminished foot pulses
—— skin shiny or discoloured
—— no hairs, thick nails
—— ulcers.
— Peripheral neuropathy — absent leg reflexes
—— diminished sensation.
— Mononeuropathy — lateral popliteal nerve — foot drop
—— III or VI — diplopia
—— muscle wasting upper leg.
— Retinopathy (see p. 85).

LOCOMOTOR SYSTEM

Normally one examines joints briefly when examining neighbouring systems. If a patient specifically complained of joint symptoms or an abnormal posture or joint is noted, more detailed examination is needed.

General habitus
• Note the following.
  — Is the patient unduly tall or short?
  — Are all limbs, spine and skull normal in size or shape?
  — Is the posture normal?
  — Curvature spine.
    Flexion: *kyphosis.*
    Extension: *lordosis.*
    Lateral: *scoliosis.*
  — Is the gait normal?
    Observing the patient walking is a vital part of examination of the locomotor system and neurological system.
    A painful gait, transferring weight quickly off a painful limb, gives an abnormal rhythm of gait.
    A painless abnormal gait may be from abnormalities of — bone
      — joint
      — muscle
      — nerve
      — or be hysterical or malingering.

Inspection

- Inspect the joints before you touch them.
- Look for:
  - enlargement
  - deformity

    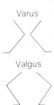

    Varus: angulation to midline.

    Valgus: angulation from midline.
  - discoloration
  - muscle wasting
- Assess whether an isolated joint is affected, or if there is polyarthritis.
- If there is polyarthritis, note if it is symmetrical or asymmetrical. Compare any abnormal findings with the other side.
  - *Arthritis* — swollen, hot, tender, painful joint.
  - *Arthropathy* — swollen but not hot and tender.
  - *Arthralgia* — painful, e.g. on movement, without being swollen. Swelling may also be due to an effusion, thickening of the periarticular tissues, enlargement of the ends of bones (e.g. *pulmonary osteopathy*) or complete disorganisation of the joint without pain (*Charcot's joint*).

Palpation

- Before you touch any joint ask the patient to tell you if it becomes painful.
- Feel for:
  - tenderness
  - warmth
  - swelling
  - fluctuation (effusion).

    An inflamed joint is usually generally tender. Localised tenderness may be mechanical in origin, e.g. ligament tear. Joint effusion may occur with an arthritis or local injury.

Movement

Test the range of movement of the joint both passively and actively. This must be done ***gently***.

- How far can the patient move the joint through its range?

    Do not seize limb and move it until patient complains.
- If range limited, can you further increase the range of movement?

Abduction: movement from central axis.

Adduction: movement to central axis.

Is the passive range of movement similar to the active range?

Limitation of the range of movement of a joint may be due to pain, muscle spasms, contracture, inflammation or thickening of the capsules or periarticular structures, effusions into the joint space, bony or cartilaginous outgrowths or painful conditions not connected with the joint

• Hold your hand round the joint whilst it is moving.   A grating or creaking sensation (*crepitus*) may be felt.

Crepitus is usually associated with osteoarthritis.

Summary of signs of common illnesses

Rheumatoid arthritis

Characteristically a polyarthritis:

— symmetrical, inflamed if active
— proximal interphalangeal and metacarpophalangeal joints of hands with ulnar deviation of fingers
— any large joint
— muscle wasting from disuse atrophy
— rheumatoid nodules on extensor surface of elbows
— may include other signs, e.g. with splenomegaly is Felty's syndrome.

Gout

Characteristically:

— asymmetrical
— inflamed first metatarsophalangeal joint (big toe) — podagra
— any joint in hand, often with tophus — hard round lump of urate by joint
— tophi on ears.

Psoriasis
- particularly involves terminal interphalangeal joints
- often with pitted nails of psoriasis as well as skin lesion.

Osteoarthritis
- 'wear and tear' of a specific joint — usually large joints
- often joints of lower limbs and asymmetrical
- Heberden's nodes — osteophytes on terminal interphalangeal joints.

Ankylosing spondylitis
- painful, stiff spine
- later fixed in flexed position
- hips and other joints can be involved.

Chapter 3
Examination of the Cardiovascular System

GENERAL EXAMINATION

- *Examine:*
  - Clubbing of finger nails.

    Clubbing in relation to the heart suggests *infective endocarditis* or *cyanotic heart disease.*
  - Cold hands with blue nails — poor perfusion, peripheral cyanosis.
  - Tongue for central cyanosis.
  - Signs of dyspnoea or distress.

    Assess the degree of breathlessness by checking if *dyspnoea* occurs on undressing, talking, at rest, or when lying flat (*orthopnoea*).

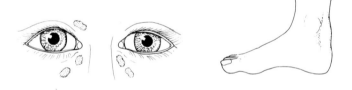

  - Xanthomata

    Xanthelasma (common) — intracutaneous yellow cholesterol deposits occur around the eyes — normal or with *hyperlipidaemia.*

    Xanthoma (uncommon).
    - *hypercholesterolaemia*
      - tendon deposits (hands and Achilles tendon)
      - tuberous xanthomas at elbows.
    - *hypertriglyceridaemia*
      - small yellow deposits on buttocks and extensor surfaces, each with a red halo.

PALPATE THE RADIAL PULSE

● *Feel the radial pulse*
> Just medial to the radius, with
> two forefingers.

Note the following:

● *Pulse rate*
> Over 15 seconds — (smart
> Alecs count for 6 seconds
> and multiply by 10).
> *Tachycardia* > 100
> *Bradycardia* < 50

● *Rhythm*
> — Regular
> > Normal variation on breathing: *sinus arrhythmia* mainly < 50
> > years.
> — Regularly irregular — pulses bigeminous, *coupled extrasystoles*
> > > (digoxin toxicity)
> > > — *Wenkebach heart block* (see ECG p. 181).
> — Irregularly irregular — *multiple extrasystoles*
> > > — *atrial fibrillation.*
> > Check apical rate by auscultation for true heart rate as small
> > pulses not transmitted to radial pulse.

● *Waveform* of the pulse
> — Normal (1).
> — Slow rising and plateau — moderate or
> severe *aortic stenosis* (2).
> — Collapsing pulse — pulse pressure
> greater than diastolic pressure,
> e.g. *aortic incompetence, elderly
> arteriosclerotic patient or gross
> anaemia* (3).
> — Bisferiens — moderate *aortic stenosis*
> with severe *incompetence* (4).
> — Pulses paradoxus — pulse weaker or
> disappears on inspiration, e.g.
> *constrictive pericarditis, tamponade,
> status asthmaticus* (5).

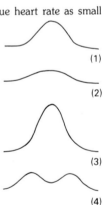

(1)

(2)

(3)

(4)

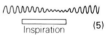
Inspiration   (5)

- *Volume*
    - Small volume — *low cardiac output.*
    - Large volume — *carbon dioxide retention*
        — *thyrotoxicosis*
        — *anaemia.*
- *Stiffness of the vessel wall*
    If stiff and tortuous, *atherosclerosis* is probably present.

TAKE THE BLOOD PRESSURE

- Wrap the cuff neatly and tightly around either upper arm.
- Gently inflate the cuff until the radial artery is no longer palpable.
- Using the stethoscope listen over the brachial artery for the pulse to appear as you drop the pressure slowly (3–4 mm/second).

- Systolic blood pressure: appearance of sounds — Korotkoff phase 1.
- Diastolic blood pressure: disappearance of sounds — Korotkoff phase 5.

Use large cuff for fat arms (circumference > 30 cm) so that inflatable cuff > ½ arm circumference.

Beware ausculatory gap with sounds disappearing mid-systole.
If sounds go to zero, use Korotkoff phase 4.

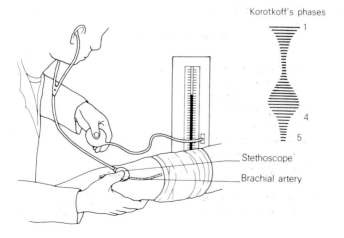

Korotkoff's phases

Stethoscope
Brachial artery

In adults, 165/95 mmHg or more is generally taken to suggest *hypertension*. The patient may be nervous when first examined and the blood pressure may be falsely high. Take it again at the end of the examination.

A wide pulse pressure (e.g. 160/30) suggests *aortic incompetence*.

A narrow pulse pressure (e.g. 95/80) suggests *aortic stenosis*.

A difference of > 20 mm systolic between arms suggests *arterial occlusion*, e.g. *dissecting aneurysm* or *atheroma*.

THE JUGULAR VENOUS PULSATION (JVP)

• *Observe the height of jugular venous pulse.*
Lie the patient down, resting at approximately 45° to the horizontal with his head on pillows, and shine a torch at an angle across the neck.
• *Look at the veins in the neck.*
   — Internal jugular vein not directly visible: pulse diffuse, medial or deep to sternomastoid.
   — External jugular vein: pulse lateral to sternomastoid. Only informative if pulsating.
• *Assess vertical height* in cm above manubriosternal angle, using pulsating external jugular vein or upper limit of internal jugular pulsation.

The *external jugular vein* is often more readily visible but may be obstructed by its tortuous course, and is less reliable than the internal jugular pulse.

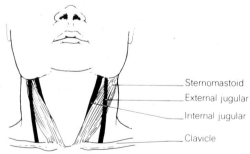

Sternomastoid

External jugular

Internal jugular

Clavicle

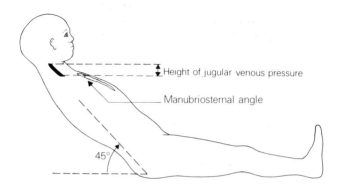

Height of jugular venous pressure

Manubriosternal angle

45°

The *internal jugular vein* is sometimes very difficult to see. Its pulsation may be confused with the cartoid artery but it — has a complex pulsation

- moves on respiration — decreases on inspiration except in tamponade
- cannot be palpated
- can be obliterated by pressure on base of neck.

The *hepatojugular reflux* is not of pathological significance but is a useful check of the level if already raised. It is elicited by pressing with the flat of the hand over the liver and watching the rise of the jugular venous pressure.

If the jugular venous pressure is found to be raised above manubriosternal angle and pulsating, it implies *right heart failure*. Do not forget to look for the other signs, i.e. pitting oedema and large tender liver. Sometimes the jugular venous pressure is so raised it can be missed except that the ears waggle.

Dilated neck veins with no pulsation suggest *non-cardiac obstruction* (e.g. carcinoma bronchus causing superior caval obstruction or kinked external jugular vein).

If the venous pressure rises on inspiration (it normally falls), *constrictive pericarditis* or pericardial effusion causing tamponade must be considered.

• *Observe the character of jugular venous pressure.*

Try to ascertain the waveform of the jugular venous pulsation. It should be a double pulsation consisting:

— 'a' wave atrial contraction — ends synchronous with carotid artery pulse 'c'
— 'v' wave atrial filling when tricuspid valve closed by ventricular contraction — with and just after carotid pulse.

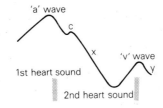

Large 'a' waves are caused by obstruction to flow from the right atrium due to stiffness of right ventricle from hypertrophy.

— Pulmonary hypertension.
— Pulmonary stenosis.
— Tricuspid stenosis.

Absent 'a' wave in atrial fibrillation.

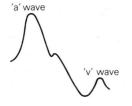

Large 'v' waves are caused by regurgitation of blood through an incompetent tricuspid valve during ventricular contraction.

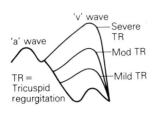

A sharp 'y' descent occurs in constrictive pericarditis.

Cannon waves (Giant 'a' waves) occur in complete heart block when the right atrium occasionally contracts against a closed tricuspid valve.

THE PRAECORDIUM

- *Inspect the praecordium for abnormal pulsation.*

    A large left ventricle will be easily seen on the left side of the chest, sometimes in the axilla.
- *Palpate the apex beat.*
  - Feel for the point furthest out and down where the pulsation can still be distinctly felt.
- *Measure the position.*
  - Which space, counting down from the second space which lies below the second rib (opposite the manubriosternal angle).
  - Laterally in centimetres from the midline.
  - Describe the apex beat in relation to the midclavicular line, anterior axillary line and midaxillary line.

    The normal position of the apex beat is fifth left intercostal space, midclavicular line.

    Try to judge if an enlarged heart is feeble (dilated) or stronger than usual (left or right ventricle hypertrophy or both).

    Thrusting displaced apex beat occurs with volume overload: an active, large stroke volume ventricle, e.g. mitral or aortic incompetence or left – right shunt.

    Sustained apex beat occurs with pressure overload: in aortic stenosis and gross hypertension. Stroke volume normal or reduced.

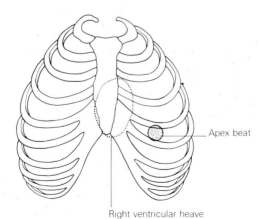

Apex beat

Right ventricular heave

Tapping apex beat (palpable first heart sound) occurs in mitral stenosis.

Diffuse pulsation asynchronous with apex beat occurs with a left ventricular aneurysm.

Impalpable — obesity, overinflated chest, pericardial effusion.

- *Palpate firmly the left border of the sternum*
  - Use the flat of your hand.

    A heave felt suggests right ventricular hypertrophy.

- *Palpate all over the praecordium* with flat of hand for thrills (palpable murmurs).

N.B. If by now you have found an abnormality in the cardiovascular system, think of possible causes before you listen.

For example, if left ventricle forceful:
- ?Hypertension — Was blood pressure (BP) raised?
- ?Aortic stenosis or incompetence — Was pulse character normal? — Will there be a murmur?
- ?Mitral incompetence — Will there be a murmur?
- ?Thyrotoxic or anaemia

AUSCULTATION

- Listen over the four main areas of the heart and in each area concentrate in order on:
  - *Heart sounds.*
  - *Added sounds.*
  - *Murmurs.*

Keep to this order when listening or describing what you have heard, or you will miss or forget important findings.

The four main areas are:
- *Apex* (and axilla if there is a murmur).
- *Tricuspid area.*
- *Aortic area* (and neck if there is a murmur).
- *Pulmonary area.*

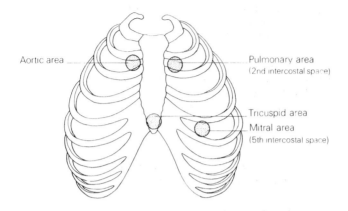

Aortic area

Pulmonary area
(2nd intercostal space)

Tricuspid area

Mitral area
(5th intercostal space)

These areas represent where one hears heart sounds and murmurs associated with these valves. They do not represent the surface markings of the valves.

If you hear little, turn the patient half left, and listen over apex (having palpated for it).

The diaphragm filters out low frequency sounds, so the bell should be used for mitral stenosis.

You may find it helpful to try to imitate what you think you hear!

Normal heart sounds

I *Sudden cessation of mitral and tricuspid flow due to valve closure.*

Loud in *mitral stenosis*.

Soft in *mitral incompetance, aortic stenosis, left bundle branch block*.

Variable in *complete heart block* and *atrial fibrillation*.

II *Sudden cessation of aortic and pulmonary flow due to valve closure* — **usually split (see below).**

Loud in *hypertension*.

Soft in *aortic* or *pulmonary stenosis*.

Wide normal split — *right bundle branch block*.
Wide fixed split — *atrial septal defect*.

Added sounds

III *Rapid ventricular filling sound in early diastole.*

>Often **normal** until about 30 years, then probably means *heart failure, fibrosed ventricle* or *constrictive pericarditis*.

IV **Atrial contraction inducing ventricular filling towards the end of the diastole.**

>May be normal but suggests increased atrial load. Not as serious a prognosis as a III heart sound.

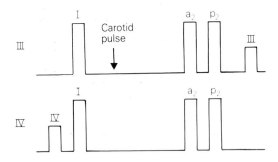

Canter rhythm (often termed *gallop*) with tachycardia gives the following cadences:

III: Tum——te—tum   or   **Ken**——tucky (k = first heart sound)
IV: te–Tum——te   or   **Te-ne**——see (n = first heart sound)

Splitting of second heart sound

Blood is drawn into the thorax during inspiration and then on to the right ventricle. There is temporarily more blood in the right ventricle than the left ventricle, and the right ventricle takes fractionally longer to empty.

Splitting is best heard during first two or three beats of inspiration. *Do not ask* patient to *hold* breath in or out when assessing splitting.

Paradoxical splitting occurs in *aortic stenosis* and *left bundle branch block*.

In both these conditions the left ventricle takes longer to empty thus

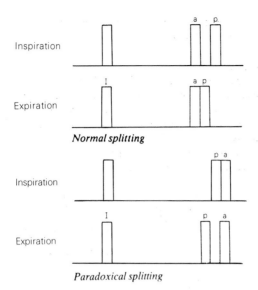

Normal splitting

Paradoxical splitting

delaying A_2 until after P_2. During inspiration P_2 occurs later and the sounds draw closer together.

Murmurs

Use the diaphragm of the stethoscope for most high pitched sounds or murmurs (e.g. aortic incompetence) and the bell for low pitched murmurs (e.g. mitral stenosis). Note the following.

- *Timing systolic or diastolic* (compare with finger on carotid pulse).
- *Site and radiation,* e.g:
    - mitral incompetence → axilla
    - aortic stenosis → carotids and apex
    - aortic incompetence → sternum.
- *Character*
    - loud or soft
    - pitch, e.g. squeaking or rumbling, 'scratchy' = pericardial or pleural
    - length — pan systolic, throughout systole
        - early diastolic, e.g. aortic or pulmonary incompetence

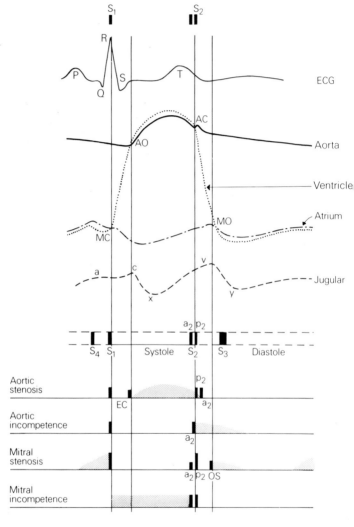

AO Aortic valve opens   MC Mitral valve closes
AC Aortic valve closes   EC Ejection click
MO Mitral valve opens   OS Opening snap

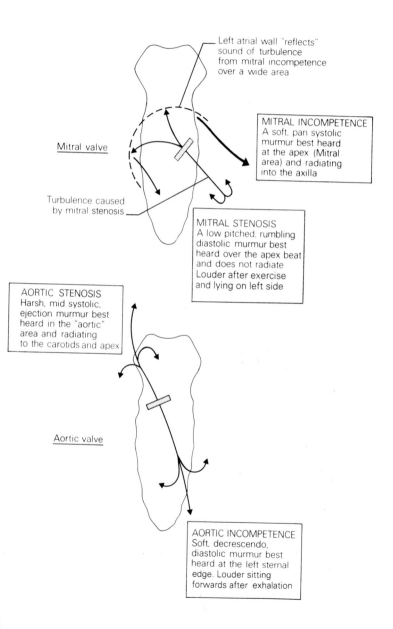

Left atrial wall "reflects" sound of turbulence from mitral incompetence over a wide area

Mitral valve

Turbulence caused by mitral stenosis

MITRAL INCOMPETENCE
A soft, pan systolic murmur best heard at the apex (Mitral area) and radiating into the axilla

MITRAL STENOSIS
A low pitched, rumbling diastolic murmur best heard over the apex beat and does not radiate. Louder after exercise and lying on left side

AORTIC STENOSIS
Harsh, mid systolic, ejection murmur best heard in the "aortic" area and radiating to the carotids and apex

Aortic valve

AORTIC INCOMPETENCE
Soft, decrescendo, diastolic murmur best heard at the left sternal edge. Louder sitting forwards after exhalation

— mid systolic, e.g. aortic stenosis or 'flow' murmur

— mid diastolic, e.g. mitral stenosis.

- *Relation to posture*
  - sit forward — aortic incompetence louder
  - lie left side — mitral stenosis louder.
- *Relation to respiration*
  - inspiration increases the murmur of a right heart lesion
  - expiration increases the murmur of a left heart lesion
  - variable — pericardial rub.
- *Relation to exercise*
  - increases the murmur of mitral stenosis.

    Diastolic murmurs are more difficult to hear than systolic murmurs.

    Ask the patient to: — lie down on his left side to hear mitral stenosis. This murmur is accentuated by mild exercise, e.g. sitting forward to touch toes six times.

    — sit forward and exhale so that aortic incompetence can be more easily heard.

N.B. Murmurs alone do not make the diagnosis. Take other signs into consideration, e.g. arterial or venous pulses, blood pressure, apex or heart sounds.

Loudness is often not proportional to severity of disease, and in some situations length of murmur is more important, e.g. mitral stenosis.

- For completion:
  - auscultate base of lungs for crepitations from left ventricular failure
  - peripheral pulses
  - palpate liver — smooth, tender, enlarged in right heart failure
  - peripheral oedema — ankle/sacral.

Summary of timing of murmurs

Ejection systolic murmur

— aortic stenosis or sclerosis (same murmur with normal pulse pressure)

- pulmonary stenosis
- atrial septal defect
- Fallot's syndrome — right outflow tract obstruction.

Pan systolic murmur
- mitral regurgitation
- tricuspid regurgitation
- ventricular septal defect.

Late systolic murmur
- mitral valve prolapse (click-murmur syndrome)
- hypertrophic cardiomyopathy
- coarction aorta (extending in diastole to a 'machinery murmur').

Early diastolic murmur
- aortic regurgitation
- pulmonary regurgitation
- Grahame–Steell murmur in pulmonary hypertension (see p. 50).

Mid–late diastolic murmur
- mitral stenosis
- tricuspid stenosis
- Austin Flint murmur in aortic incompetence (see p. 50)
- left atrial myxoma (variable — can also give other murmurs).

SIGNS OF LEFT AND RIGHT VENTRICULAR FAILURE

Left heart failure
- Look for the following.
  - Dyspnoea.
  - Basal crepitations.
  - Fourth heart sound or third in older patients.
- Sit the patient forward and listen at the bases of the lungs with the diaphragm of the stethoscope for fine crepitations.

> Fine crepitations are caused by alveoli opening an inspiration. When a patient has been recumbent for a while, alveoli tend to collapse in the normal lung. On taking a deep breath

crepitations will be heard but do not mean pulmonary oedema. Ask the patient to cough. If crepitations continue after this, pulmonary oedema may be present.

Right heart failure
- Look for the following.
    - Raised jugular venous pressure.
    - Enlarged tender liver (see later).
    - Pitting oedema.
- With the patient sitting forward look for swelling over the sacral area. If there is, push your thumb into the swelling and see if you leave an indentation. If you do, this is called pitting oedema.
- Check both ankles for pitting oedema.

> Oedema (fluid) collects at the most dependent part of the body. A patient who is mostly sitting will have ankle oedema while a patient who is lying will have predominantly sacral oedema.

FUNCTIONAL RESULT

- Having ascertained the basic pathology (e.g. myocardial infarction, aortic stenosis, pericarditis), make an assessment of the functional result
    - *History.* How far can the patient walk, etc.
    - *Examination.* Evidence of — cardiac enlargement (hypertrophy or dilatation)
        - heart failure
        - arrhythmias
        - pulmonary hypertension
        - cyanosis
        - endocarditis.
    - *Investigations.* For example — chest X-ray
        - ECG
        - treadmill exercise test with ECG for ischaemia
        - echocardiograph — sonar 'radar' of heart, for muscle and ventricle size, contractility, valve function (particularly mitral valve)

- 24 hour ECG tape for arrythmias
- Cardiac catheterisation for pressure measurements, blood oxygenation and angiogram
- Radioactive scan — to image live, ischaemic or dead cardiac muscle.

SUMMARY OF SIGNS OF COMMON ILLNESSES

Mitral stenosis
- Small pulse — fibrillating?
- JVP only raised if heart failure.
- RV++ LVo Tapping apex.
- Loud I. Loud P_2 if pulmonary hypertension.
- Opening snap (os). Mid diastolic murmur at apex only (low pitched rumbling). Severity indicated by early os and long murmur.
- Pre systolic accentuation murmur (absent if atrial fibrillation and stiff cusps).
- Sounds 'ta ta rooofoo T'
  from   'II os murmur I'

Mitral incompetence
- Fibrillating?
- JVP only raised if heart failure.
- RV+ LV++ Systolic thrill.
- Soft I. Loud P_2 if pulmonary hypertension.
- Pan systolic murmur apex → axilla.
       Mitral valve prolapse.
       Mid systolic click, late systolic murmur.
       Posterior cusp — apex → axilla.
       Anterior cusp — apex → aortic area.

Aortic stenosis
- Plateau pulse — narrow pulse pressure.
- JVP only raised if heart failure.

— LV+ +   Systolic thrill.
— Soft A_2 with paradoxical split ($\pm$ ejection click).
— Harsh mid systolic murmur, apex and base radiating to carotids.
— Note discrepancy of forceful apex and feeble atrial pulse.

Aortic incompetence
— Water hammer pulse — wide pulse pressure. Pulse visible in carotids.
— JVP only raised if heart failure.
— LV+ + with dilation.
— (Ejection click).
— Early diastolic murmur base $\rightarrow$ lower sternum (also ejection systolic murmur from increased flow).
— (Sometimes Austin Flint murmur — see below).

Austin Flint murmur
— Mid diastolic murmur (like mitral stenosis) in aortic incompetence due to regurgitant stream of blood on anterior cusp mitral valve.

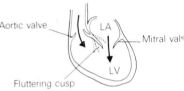

Graham–Steell murmur
— Pulmonary early diastolic murmur (functional PI) in mitral stenosis or other causes of pulmonary hypertension.

Atrial septal defect
— JVP only raised if failure or tricuspid incompetence.
— RV+ + LVo.
— Widely fixed split second sound.
— Pulmonary systolic murmur (tricuspid diastolic flow murmur).

Ventricular septal defect
— RV+ LV+ .
— Pan systolic murmur left sternal edge (loud if small defect!).

Patent ductus arteriosus
— Systolic → diastolic 'machinery' or continuous murmur below left clavicle.

Metal prosthetic valves
— loud clicks with short flow murmur — aortic systolic
— mitral diastolic.

Pericardial rub
— Scratchy, superficial noise heard in systole and diastole.
— Brought out by stethoscope pressure, and sometimes variable with respiration.

Infectious endocarditis
— Febrile, unwell, anaemia.
— Clubbing.
— Splinter haemorrhages.
— Osler's nodes.
— Cardiac murmur.
— Splenomegaly.

Rheumatic fever
— Flitting arthralgia.
— Erythema nodosum or erythema marginatum.
— Tachycardia.
— Murmurs.
— Sydenham's chorea.

Clues to diagnosis from facial appearance
— Down's syndrome — ventricular septal defect
— patent ductus arteriosus.
— Marfan's syndrome — aortic regurgitation.
— Turner's syndrome — coarctation.
— Thyrotoxicosis — atrial fibrillation.

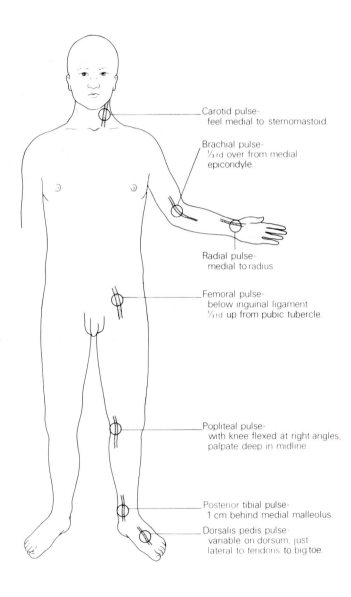

Carotid pulse-
feel medial to sternomastoid.

Brachial pulse-
⅓rd over from medial
epicondyle.

Radial pulse-
medial to radius

Femoral pulse-
below inguinal ligament
⅓rd up from pubic tubercle.

Popliteal pulse-
with knee flexed at right angles,
palpate deep in midline.

Posterior tibial pulse-
1 cm behind medial malleolus.

Dorsalis pedis pulse-
variable on dorsum, just
lateral to tendons to big toe.

PERIPHERAL PULSES

• Feel all peripheral pulses. Leg pulses are usually felt after examining the abdomen.

> Diminished or absent pulses suggest blockages — atheroma.
>
> The leg pulses are particularly important if there is a history of intermittent claudication.
>
> *Auscultation* of the carotid and femoral vessels is useful if there is a suspicion these arteries are partially blocked. A *bruit* is easily heard if the partial blockage causes turbulence of flow.
>
> *Coarctation* of the aorta delays the femoral pulse after the radial pulse.

VARICOSE VEINS

• Varicose veins and herniae (see p. 72) are examined when the patient is standing, possibly at the end of the whole examination at the same time as the gait (see p. 103).

> Majority due to incompetent valves in long saphenous vein or short saphenous vein.
>
> Long saphenous — from femoral vein in groin to medial side of lower leg.
>
> Short saphenous — from popliteal fossa to back of calf and lateral malleolus.

• Observe
  - swelling
  - pigmentation
  - eczema
  - inflammation.
• Palpate
  - soft or hard (thrombosed)
  - tender — 'thrombophlebitis'
  - cough impulse — implies incompetent valves.
    > Incompetent valves can be tested by the *Trendelenberg test:*
    > - Elevate leg to empty veins.
    > - Apply pressure in groin over long saphenous vein (with finger or cuff).

— Stand patient. If veins stay empty, until you release groin pressure, the incompetence is at the groin.

If veins fill immediately on standing, then incompetent valves are in thigh or calf, so do the *Perthes test:*

— As for Trendelenberg, but on standing let some blood enter veins by temporary release of groin pressure.

— Ask patient to stand up and down on toes.

— Veins become less tense if : — muscle pump is satisfactory
  — perforating calf veins are patent with competent valves.

Chapter 4
Examination of the Chest

GENERAL INSPECTION

- Examine the patient for:
  - nicotine on fingers
  - clubbing
    - Respiratory causes include: — *carcinoma of bronchus*
      - *mesothelioma*
      - *bronchiectasis*
      - *lung abscess*
      - *empyema*
      - *fibrosing alveolitis.*
  - evidence of respiratory failure
    - Hypoxia — central cyanosis
    - Hypercapnia — drowsy, confusion, papilloedema
      - warm hands, bounding pulse, dilated veins
      - coarse tremor/flap.
  - respiratory rate — count per minute
  - pattern of respiration
    - Cheyne Stokes — alternating hyperventilation and apnoea
      - severe increased intracranial pressure
      - left ventricular failure
      - high altitude.
  - obstructive airways disease
    - Pursed lip breathing — expiration against partially closed lips
      - chronic obstructive airways disease to delay closure of bronchioles.
    - Use of accessory muscles — sternomastoids
      - strap muscles and platysmus.
  - wheezing
  - stridor — partial obstruction of major airway
  - hoarse voice — abnormal vocal chords
    - or recurrent laryngeal palsy.

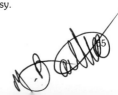

First examine the front of the chest fully and then similarly examine the back of the chest

INSPECTION OF THE CHEST

- Rest the patient comfortably in the bed at 45°.
  - — grossly distended neck, puffy blue face and arms.
    Superior mediastinal obstruction.
- Inspect the *shape* of the chest.
  - — Asymmetry: diminution of one side.
    Lung collapse.
    Fibrosis.
  - — Deformity: check spine.
  - — Pectus excavatum: sunken sternum.
  - — Barrel chest: lower costal recession on deep inspiration. Cricoid cartilage close to sternal notch. Chest appears to be fixed in 'inspiration' — *obstructive airways disease.*

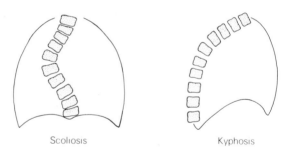

Scoliosis   Kyphosis

PALPATION

- Mediastinum position.
  - — Check position of the *trachea*. Palpate with a single finger in the midline and determine if it slips preferentially to one side or the other.
  - — *Lymph nodes* supraclavicular fossae — *TB, cancer bronchus.*

— *Apex beat.* This may be displaced because of enlarged heart and not a shift in the mediastinum.

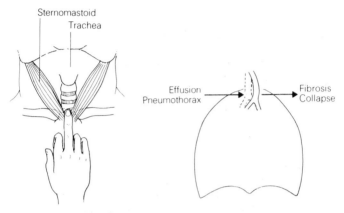

- Unequal movement of chest.
  - Look from the end of the bed.
  - Lay a hand comfortably on either side of the chest and using these as a gauge, assess if there is diminution of one side during inspiration.

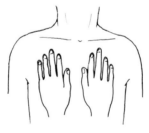

Diminution of movement on one side indicates pathology on that side.

PERCUSSION

- Percuss with the middle finger of one hand against the middle phalanx of the middle finger of the other laid flat on the chest. The finger should strike at right angles.

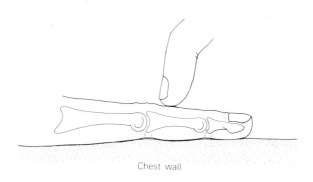

Chest wall

• Percuss both sides of the chest for resonance, at top, middle and lower segments. Compare sides, and if abnormal also compare the front and back of chest.
• If a dull area exists, map out its limits by percussing from a resonant to the dull area.
• Percuss the level of the diaphragm from above downwards.

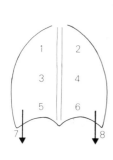

Increased resonance may occur in
— *pneumothorax.*
— *emphysema.*
Decreased resonance may occur in
— *effusion: stony* dullness.
— *solid lung* — consolidation
              — collapse
              — abscess
              — neoplasm.
Remember the surface markings of the lungs when percussing.
Thus the lower lobe predominates posteriorly and the upper lobe predominates anteriorly.

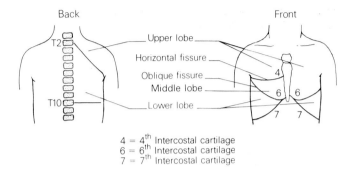

4 = 4th Intercostal cartilage
6 = 6th Intercostal cartilage
7 = 7th Intercostal cartilage

AUSCULTATION

• Before listening, ask patient to cough up any sputum which may provide noises for bronchi.
• Use the bell of the stethoscope and listen at the top, middle and bottom of both sides of the chest, and then in the axilla. Ask the patient to breathe through his mouth moderately deeply. It helps to demonstrate this yourself.

> The stethoscope diaphragm is less effective if the patient is thin with prominent ribs or if the chest is hairy.

• Listen for *breath sounds*, comparing both sides.
  — Vesicular: normal breath sound (1)

  Inspiration Expiration

  — Bronchial: patent bronchi plus conducting tissue (2)
    Consolidation (usually pneumonia).

    Inspiration Expiration

    Neoplasm.
    Fibrosis.
    Abscess
    Not collapse, effusion (except occasionally at surface).

— Diminution: indicates either no air movement (e.g. obstructed bronchus) or air or fluid preventing sound conduction.

  Effusion.

  Pneumothorax.

  Emphysema.

  Collapse.

- Listen for *added sounds*, and note if inspiratory or expiratory.
  — Pleural rub.

    Caused by *pleurisy* (inflammation due to infection or infarction), but make sure it does not come from friction of skin or hairs against stethoscope.
  — Ronchi or wheezing.

    Constricted air passages giving dry tubular sounds, often maximal on expiration.
  — Râles or crepitations or crackles.

    Fine — *heart failure*
       — *alveolitis*.

    Medium — *infection*.

    Coarse — air bubbling through fluid in larger bronchioles, e.g. *bronchiectasis*. If relieved by coughing, suggests from bronchioles.

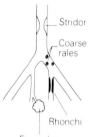

Stridor

Coarse rales

Rhonchi

Fine rales

VOCAL RESONANCE

Normally only if pathology is suspected, but you must practice to become familiar with normal resonance.

Note that alteration of breath sounds and vocal resonance depend on the same criteria and alter together.

- Ask the patient to repeat '99' whilst listening to chest in the same areas as auscultation. The sounds are louder over areas of consolidation. Compare both sides.

    At the surface of an *effusion* the words '99' take on a bleating character like a goat, which is called *aegophony*. If vocal resonance gross, *whispering pectoriloquy* can be elicited by asking the patient to whisper '1, 2, 3, 4'.

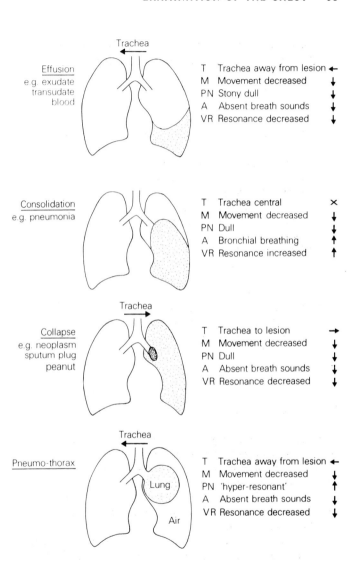

Trachea

Effusion
e.g. exudate
transudate
blood

T   Trachea away from lesion ←
M   Movement decreased   ↓
PN Stony dull   ↓
A   Absent breath sounds   ↓
VR Resonance decreased   ↓

Consolidation
e.g. pneumonia

T   Trachea central   ×
M   Movement decreased   ↓
PN Dull   ↓
A   Bronchial breathing   ↑
VR Resonance increased   ↑

Trachea

Collapse
e.g. neoplasm
sputum plug
peanut

T   Trachea to lesion   →
M   Movement decreased   ↓
PN Dull   ↓
A   Absent breath sounds   ↓
VR Resonance decreased   ↓

Trachea

Pneumo-thorax

Lung

Air

T   Trachea away from lesion ←
M   Movement decreased   ↓
PN 'hyper-resonant'   ↑
A   Absent breath sounds   ↓
VR Resonance decreased   ↓

N.B. — vocal fremitus, breath sounds, vocal resonance all depend on same criteria and vary together.

- To determine further clues check:
  - chest movement asymmetry
  - mediastinum displacement
  - percussion.

SPUTUM

Examination of the sputum is unpleasant but important.
- Look for:
  - quantity (increased grossly in bronchiectasis)
  - consistency (if all mucous it may be saliva)
  - colour (if yellow or green it may be infected)
  - blood (cancer, TB, embolus).
    Ideally the sputum should be examined under the microscope
    for — bacteria
      - pus cells
      - eosinophils
      - plugs
      - asbestos.

FUNCTIONAL RESULT

- Make an assessment of the functional result.
  - *History.* How far can the patient walk, etc.
  - *Examination.* $P_{O_2}\downarrow$ — central cyanosis
    — confusion.
    $P_{CO_2}\uparrow$ — peripheral signs — warm periphery
      — dilated veins
      — bounding pulse
      — flapping tremor.
    — central signs — drowsy
      — papilloedema
      — small pupils.
    — check by arterial blood gases.

— *Tests* (usually of obstructive airways disease):

At the bedside: Blowing out a lighted match about 15 cm from the mouth and with the mouth wide open is easy as long as your peak flow is above approximately 80 litre/min (normal 300–500 litre/min).

Expiration time: An assessment of airways obstruction can be made by timing the period of full expiration through wide open mouth following a deep breath. This should be less than 2 seconds in the normal.

Chest expansion: Expansion from full inspiration to a full expiration should be more than 5 cm. Reduced if hyperinflation of the chest due to chronic obstructive airways disease.

Peak flow meter: A measure of airways obstruction is the peak rate of flow of air out of the lungs. A record is made using a machine. Normal 300–500 litre/min.

SUMMARY OF COMMON ILLNESSES

Asthma
— patient distressed, tachypnoeic, unable to talk easily
— wheeze audible or on auscultation
— over-inflated chest with hyper-resonance
— if central cyanosis: critically ill, artifical ventilation?
— pulsus paradoxus (may be normal between attacks).

Obstructive airways disease (chronic)
— barrel chest
— accessory muscles of respiration in use
— hyper-resonance
— depressed diaphragm — indrawing lower costal margin on inspiration
— diminished breath sounds.

    Blue Bloater — central cyanosis
            — signs of CO_2 retention
            — obese
            — not dyspnoeic
            — ankle oedema: may or may not have right heart failure.

Pink Puffer — not cyanosed
— no CO_2 retention
— thin
— dyspnoeic
— no oedema.

Bronchiectasis

— clubbing
— constant green/yellow phlegm
— coarse râles over affected area.

Allergic alveolitis

— clubbing
— fine, unexplained râles, widespread over bases.

Chapter 5
Examination of the Abdomen

GENERAL INSPECTION

- Look for signs of:
  - chronic liver disease: — *clubbing*
    - *leuconychia*
    - *palmar erythema*
    - *telangiectasia on face*
    - *spider naevi*
    - *icterus*
    - *gynaecomastia*
    - *Dupuytren's contraction.*

Spider naevus
A small collection of capillaries fed by a central arteriole

  - liver failure: — *liver flap*
    - *faetor hepaticus*
    - *confusion.*

    Signs of chronic liver disease are usually obvious, but we are all allowed up to six spider naevi (particularly if pregnant!).
  - check for anaemia.
  - Fe deficiency: — *koilonychia*
    - *smooth tongue*
    - *angular stomatitis* — can be from ill fitting dentures or oedentulous.

Virchow's node

  - palpate for nodes behind the left sternoclavicular joint.

    A hard node felt behind the left sternoclavicular joint is *Virchow's Node* (he diagnosed this on himself) and suggests an abdominal neoplasm.
- Look at mouth:
  - *dry tongue* — 'dehydration' or mouth breathing

    If patient seems dehydrated lift fold of skin on neck. Remains raised with dehydration and old age.

— *monilia* — red tongue, white patches on palate
— *gingivitis*
— teeth
— breath — *ketosis, ethanol, faetor hepaticus* and *uraemia.*

INSPECTION OF THE ABDOMEN

• Lie the patient flat (one pillow) with arms by his sides.
• Expose the abdomen from chest margin to groin.

In an exam, stand back to look at the abdomen, so the examiner is impressed you are inspecting before palpating!

• Look for:
— skin — striae: pink in *Cushing's syndrome*
— body hair
— nodules
— surgical scars
— swelling — central or flank
— symmetrical or asymmetrical

    Flatus.
    Faeces.
    Foetus.
    Fat.
    Fluid (ascites, ovarian cyst).
— movement: on respiration
— peristalsis: may be visible in thin normal person
— pulsation
— hernia
— dilated veins — flow of blood in vein is:
    Superior: due to inferior vena cava obstruction.
    Inferior: due to superior vena cava obstruction.
    Radiating from navel: due to portal vein
    obstruction.

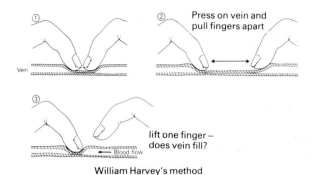

William Harvey's method

Describe findings using these descriptions:

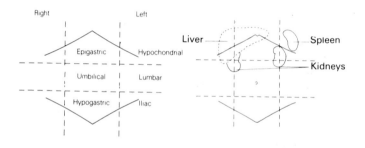

PALPATE THE ABDOMEN

• Palpate the groins for enlarged lymph nodes. (If you don't do it now, you may forget later!)

> Most people have small, shotty nodes. Most enlarged tender nodes arise from infection in legs or feet.
>
> If large nodes, palpate spleen carefully (reticulosis or leukaemia).

Before you feel abdomen

• Ask: 'Is your tummy painful anywhere?' 'Tell me if I hurt you.'

- Have warm hands, and the patient lying flat.
- Lightly palpate each quadrant first, starting away from the site of pain or tenderness. The hand should be flat on the abdomen and feel with fingers flexed at the metacarpophalangeal joints. Be gentle.
- *Look at the patient's face* to see if palpation is hurting him.

> *Tenderness* may be superficial, deep, or rebound.

> *Rebound tenderness* is produced by rapid removal of deep palpation and may occur in peritonitis.

> *Guarding* may be noted during palpation. This is a reflex action to protect from pain.

> *Rigidity.* Fixed, tense abdominal muscles. Occurs in generalised peritonitis.

PALPATION OF THE ORGANS

Liver

- Palpate with fingers flexed at metacarpophalangeal joints, using side of forefinger parallel with liver, with the patient breathing moderately deeply. Start about 10 cm below the costal margin and work up towards the ribs.
- Describe position of liver edge in centimetres below the costal margin of midclavicular line. Feel edge for:
  — texture
  — regular/irregular
  — tender
  — pulsatile (in tricuspid incompetence).
- Percuss the upper and lower borders of liver after palpation to confirm findings.

> If the liver is not felt and the right hypochondrium is dull the liver may extend to the hypogastrium! Palpate lower down.

If the liver is large describe.

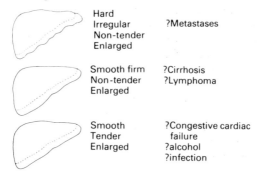

Hard
Irregular   ?Metastases
Non-tender
Enlarged

Smooth firm   ?Cirrhosis
Non-tender   ?Lymphoma
Enlarged

Smooth   ?Congestive cardiac
Tender   failure
Enlarged   ?alcohol
               ?infection

If large remember to feel for the spleen.

Spleen

• As for the liver, palpate 10 cm beneath the costal margin in the hypochondrium, working up to ribs.
• Ask the patient to take a deep breath, to bring spleen down so it can be palpated.
• If the spleen is not palpable, check the area for splenic dullness by percussion — the spleen can be enlarged to the hypogastrium!
    If a slightly enlarged spleen is suspected, lie the patient on the right side with the left arm hanging loosely in front and again feel on deep inspiration.
• Characteristics of the spleen:
    — site
    — shape (?notch)
    — cannot get above it
    — moves on respiration
    — dull to percussion.
Describe as for liver.

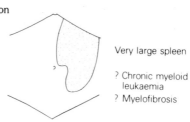

Very large spleen

? Chronic myeloid
  leukaemia
? Myelofibrosis

Kidneys

- Palpate bimanually.
- Push up with left hand in renal angle and feel kidney anteriorly with right hand.
- Ask the patient to take a deep breath to bring kidneys between hands.
  Tenderness is common over the kidneys if there is infection. A large kidney may indicate a tumour, polycystic disease, or hydronephrosis.

Masses

- Carefully palpate the whole of the abdomen. If a mass is found, describe:
  - site
  - size
  - shape
  - consistency — faeces may be indented by pressure
  - fixation or mobility — does it move on respiration?
  - tender
  - pulsatile — transmitted pulsation from aorta or pulsatile swelling
  - dull to percussion — particularly important to determine if bowel in front of mass
  - does it alter after defaecation or micturition?

Aorta

- Palpate in the midline above the umbilicus for a pulsatile mass. If easily palpated:
  - it may be normal in a thin person
  - unfolded aorta
  - aneurysm large — expansile — bruit.

PERCUSSION

Only percuss the abdomen if there is an abnormal finding, e.g. a mass or swelling.

- If there is generalised swelling of the abdomen, lie the patient on one side and mark the upper level of dullness. Roll the patient to the other side and see if the level shifts. This is called shifting dullness.

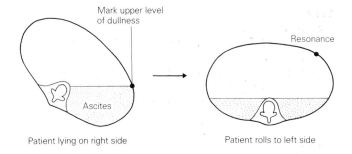

Mark upper level of dullness

Resonance

Ascites

Patient lying on right side

Patient rolls to left side

AUSCULTATION

Bowel sounds

Listen for bowel sounds only if there is an abnormal finding, e.g. abdominal pain. Listen over the abdomen with the diaphragm of the stethoscope for about 10–15 seconds.

> *Obstruction* of the bowel gives hyperactive bowel sounds or 'tinkling'
>
> *Paralytic* ileus gives complete absence of bowel sounds.

Arterial bruits

If appropriate from the history or examination (e.g. hypertension), listen for bruits over the renal or femoral arteries.

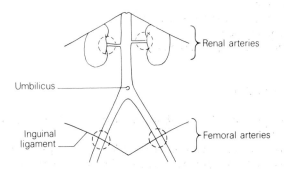

Renal arteries

Umbilicus

Inguinal ligament

Femoral arteries

Renal artery stenosis may be the cause of hypertension.

Patients with *intermittent claudication* may have atheromatous bruits over the femoral arteries.

Listen for *hepatic bruits* in patients with liver disease.

HERNIAE

• Establish the appropriate anatomical landmarks — pubic tubercle, anterior superior iliac spine, femoral artery.

• Examine the patient lying down and ask him to cough. An abnormal pulse suggests a hernia.

• Stand the patient up, re-examine with the patient coughing if you are not to miss a small hernia.

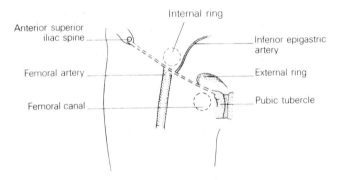

Indirect (oblique) inguinal hernia: swelling reduced to internal inguinal ring by pressure on contents of hernial sac and then controlled by pressure over the internal ring when patient asked to cough. If hand is then removed, impulses passes medially towards external ring and is palpable **above and medial** to pubic tubercle.

   Direct inguinal hernia: impulse in a forward direction *medial to femoral artery* and swelling not controlled by pressure over internal ring.

   Fermoral hernia: swelling **below and lateral** to pubic tubercle, emerging from femoral canal.

EXAMINATION OF GENITALS

• In the male palpate the scrotum for the testes and epididymes. It is rarely necessary to examine the penis.

Tender and enlarged testes may occur with *orchitis* or *torsion of the testis*.

A *large, hard, painless testis suggests cancer*.

A large, soft swelling which transilluminates suggests *hydrocoele*.

Balanitis (inflamed glans of penis) must remind the examiner to check for diabetes.

PER RECTUM EXAMINATION

Never perform a rectal examination without permission from the houseman or registrar, or without a chaperone for female patients.
• Tell the patient at each stage what you are going to do.
• Lie the patient on the left side with knees flexed to the chest.
• Say 'I am going to put a finger into your back passage'.
• Inspect anus for haemorrhoids and fissures.
• With lubricant on glove, gently insert forefinger into rectum. Feel the tone of the sphinter, size and character of the prostate and any lateral masses. If appropriate proceed to proctoscopy.
• Test stool on your glove for occult blood.

PER VAGINAL EXAMINATION

Never perform a vaginal examination without a chaperone, female if possible, and only on the direction of a qualified instructor.
• Tell the patient at each stage what you are going to do.
• Lie the patient on her left side as for per rectal examination (although some physicians prefer patient lying on back with hips flexed and abducted).
• Inspect the external genitalia.
• With lubricant on glove insert one finger into vagina and then a second finger if there is room.
• Palpate the cervix.

- Examine for position and enlargement of uterus, tenderness of appendages and masses.
- Check for discharge by observing glove.

SUMMARY OF SIGNS IN COMMON ILLNESS

Cirrhosis
— white nails
— clubbing
— liver palms
— spider naevi
— jaundice
— firm liver.

Portal hypertension
— splenomegaly
— ascites
— caput medusa.

Hepatic encephalopathy
— liver flap
— drowsy
— constructional apraxia (cannot draw five-pointed star)
— musty foetor.

'Dehydration' (water and salt loss)
— dry skin
— veins collapsed
— diminished skin turgor — pinched fold of skin remains raised
— tongue dry
— eyes sunken
— blood pressure low with postural drop.

Intestinal obstruction
— patient 'dehydrated' if has been vomiting
— abdomen centrally swelling
— visible peristalsis
— not tender (unless inflammation, or some other pathology)

- resonant to percussion
- loud 'tinkling' bowel sounds.

Pyloric stenosis
- upper abdomen swelling
- may have 'succussion splash' on shaking abdomen
- otherwise like intestinal obstruction.

Appendicitis
- slight fever
- deep tenderness right iliac fossa or per rectum
- otherwise little to find unless has spread to peritonitis.

Peritonitis
- lies still
- abdomen — does not move on respiration
    - rigid on palpation (guarding)
    - tender, particularly on removing fingers rapidly (rebound tenderness)
    - absent bowel sounds.

Cholecystitis
- tender right hypochondrium, particularly on breathing in (Murphy's sign — tender gall bladder descends on inspiration to touch your palpating hand).

Jaundice and palpable gall bladder
- obstruction is not due to gall stones, but from another obstruction such as neoplasm pancreas (Courvoisier's Law). Gall stones have usually caused a fibrosed gall bladder which cannot dilate from back pressure from gallstones in common bile duct.

Enlarged spleen
- infective e.g. septicaemia or subacute bacterial endocarditis
- portal hypertension, e.g. cirrhosis
- lymphoma
- leukaemia and other haematological diseases
- auto-immune, e.g. systemic lupus, Felty's syndrome.

Chapter 6
Examination of the Nervous System

The history is of prime importance in assessing the nature of the pathology, whereas the examination reveals the localisation and extent of the lesion. The following features in the history can be informative:

— speed of onset — rapid — vascular or infective

— slow, progressive — neoplasm or degenerative disorder

— remittant — mechanical, obstruction or pressure

— demyelination, e.g. *multiple sclerosis*

— brief episodes with recovery — epilepsy, vascular migraine, syncope.

The minute examination of the nervous system can be elaborated almost indefinitely. Of far greater importance is to acquire the ability to conduct a thorough but comparatively rapid examination with confidence in the findings.

From the history it will usually be obvious whether it is necessary to examine the higher cerebral functions in detail. A patient with sciatica would rightly be dismayed by an examination which began by asking him to name the parts of a watch. The order in which functions are examined may be varied according to the symptoms, but the routine examination must be mastered.

The examination of the nervous system is approached under the following headings.

Higher cerebral function.

Cranial nerves.

Limbs and trunk
- general inspection
- arms
- trunk
- legs
- sensation
- gait.

The nervous system cannot be examined in isolation. Other points of relevance may include:
— blood pressure
— heart, e.g. arrhythmia, mitral stenosis
— carotid arteries — palpation and bruit
— configuration of the skull and spine
— neck stiffness
— ear drums for otitis media.

HIGHER CEREBRAL FUNCTIONS

General observation
• Appearance, e.g. unkempt.
• Behaviour, e.g. bewildered, restless, agitated.
• Emotional state, e.g. depressed, euphoric, hostile.

Conscious level
If the patient is not fully conscious:
• Shake him gently or speak to him loudly.
    Record:
        Drowsy but rousable to normal level.
        Drowsy but not rousable.
If the patient does not respond and is apparently unconscious:
• Assess his response to a painful stimulus, e.g. twist fold of skin, rub patient's ribs with your knuckles.
    Record:
        Semi-purposeful movement to pain, e.g. as if to brush away obnoxious stimulus.
        Reflex movements to pain, e.g. extends limbs.
        No response to pain.
It may be useful to ask ward staff for their observations.

Mood
• If evidence for depression, worry, agitation or irritability, record current nature and severity.

Confusion
• If a patient appears confused, move on to assess cognitive state including disorientation.

Speech
Assess from conversation.
• Is there difficulty in articulation?
If necessary, ask patient to say 'British Constitution', 'West Register Street'.

— *Dysarthria* — cerebellar — scanning or staccato.

— extra pyramidal
— lower motor neurone
— upper motor neurone
— acute alcohol poisoning
} — slurred.

• Is there altered voice tone?
— *Dysphonia* — cord lesion — hoarse.
— hysterical
— palatal palsy — nasal.
• Is there difficulty in finding the right word?
— *Dysphasia or aphasia* — disorder of use of words as symbols in speech, writing and understanding. Nearly always due to left hemiphere lesion.
    N.B. Right or left-handed? May be right lesion if left handed.
— *Slight dysphasia* — difficult to detect. Mispronounced words and circumlocutions in spontaneous speech. Test for *nominal aphasia* by asking patient to name objects you point to, e.g. wristwatch, pen, tie. Understanding seems intact.
— *Gross dysphasia* — usually obvious. Spontaneous speech scanty, small vocabulary, often with wrong words used.
— *Aphasia* — no speech at all, just grunts.

Other defects occurring in absence of motor or sensory dysfunction
— *Dyslexia* — inappropriate difficulty with reading. Read few lines from newspaper (having established that comprehension and expressive speech are intact).

— *Dysgraphia* — loss of ability to write.

— *Acalculia* — loss of ability to do mental and written sums.

— *Apraxia* — inability to perform a purposeful task when no motor or sensory loss, e.g. opening matchbox, waving goodbye. Apraxia for dressing common in diffuse brain disease. Inability to draw five-pointed star occurs in hepatic pre-coma.

— *Agnosia* — inability to recognise objects (e.g. a key or coin when placed in hand. Tactile agnosia = astereognosis).

— *Parietal lobe lesions* — especially right, cause spatial difficulties; getting lost in familiar places, inability to lay table or draw or make patterns with matches, neglect of left side of space, or of half of body.

Flow, form and content of speech

- Rate and quantity
    - fast in mania, slow in depression. Often little spontaneous speech in dementia.
- Form
    - are there abnormalities of grammar and flow? Record an example. Disordered thought processes can occur in *schizophrenia*, *mania*, *acute organic states*, *dementia*.
- Content
    - delusions — false, unshakeable belief, e.g. I've got syphilis/cancer.
    - obsessions — intrusive thoughts or repetitious behaviour which the patient cannot resist although he knows they are not sensible.
    - perseveration — repetition of a word or phrase.
    - illusions — misinterpreted perceptions, e.g. he thinks you are a policeman. Common in acute organic state (*psychosis*).
    - hallucinations — false perception, e.g. pink elephants. Can be visual or auditory and occur in acute organic states, dementia, schizophrenia and mania. Can be auditory or visual.

Cognitive

Take account of any evidence you have about the patient's intelligence, education and interests.

Orientation
- Awareness of:
  - time: 'What day is it?' (time, month, year).
  - place: Where are you?'
  - person: What is your name?'

    Disorientation suggests acute organic state or dementia.

    Depressed patients may be unwilling to reply although they know the answers.

Attention and calculation
- Test the concentration of a patient by asking him to take away 7 from 100, 7 from 93, etc., or by asking him to say the months of the year backwards.

    Concentration may be impaired with many cerebral abnormalities, depression and anxiety.

Memory
Immediate recall — digit span.
- Repeat digits spoken slowly. Start with easy short sequence and then increase the numbers. Most people manage 7 digits forwards, 5 backwards.

Short-term memory.
- Ask patient to tell you:
  - what he had for breakfast
  - what he did the night before
  - what he has read in today's paper.

    Demented patients will be unable to do this. They may confabulate (make up impressive stories) to cover their ignorance.

New memory
- Give a name and address, make sure the patient has learnt it, and then test recall at 5 minutes.

Longer-term memory
- Ask patient:
  - for events before illness, e.g. last year, or during last week
  - what is your address?

General knowledge

Assess in relation to anticipated performance from history.

- What is the name of the Queen (Prime Minister)?
- Name six capital cities.
- What were the dates of the last war?

> In *acute organic states and dementia*, new learning, recent memory and reasoning are usually more impaired than remote memory. Vocabulary is usually well preserved in dementia. A history from relative or employer is very important in early dementia. In depression, patients may be unwilling to reply, and appear demented.

Reasoning — abstract thought

- What does this proverb mean 'Let sleeping dogs lie?'

Ward behaviour

- Observe for yourself, and ask for nurse's and relative's comments on patient's awareness, self care, etc.

SKULL AND SPINE

- Inspect and palpate skull if any possibility of a head injury.
- Neck stiffness — meningeal irritation (see p. 106)
- Spine — inspect, usually when examining back of chest.
- If any possibility of pathology, stand patient, and check all movements of spine.

CRANIAL NERVES

- Examine cranial nerves and upper limbs with patient sitting up, preferable on side of bed or on a chair.

I Olfactory

Not normally tested unless other neurological defects including papilloedema, undiagnosed headache or head injury.

> Oil of cloves, peppermint, coffee, etc, each nostril in turn.

> It is normal not to be able to name smells, but one smell should be distinguished from another.

Pungent or noxious smells such as ammonia should not be used, as they are perceived by the V cranial nerve.

Abnormal — rhinitis
— base skull fracture
— olfactory groove meningioma.

II Optic

Visual acuity
- Ask patient to read small newspaper print with each eye separately.
- If sight poor, test formally:
  - near vision — newsprint or Jaeger type (each eye in turn).
  - distant vision — Snellen's type (more precise method).

    Stand patient at 6 metres from Snellen's card (each eyes in turn).

    Results expressed:

    6 — distance of person from card.

    x — distance at which should be able to read type.

    i.e. 6/6 is good vision, 6/60 means the smallest type patient can read is large enough to be normally read to 60 metres.

    If cannot read 6/6, try with correction with glasses or pinhole.
    Looking through a pinhole in a card obviates refractive errors, analogous to a pinhole camera. If vision remains poor suspect a neurological or ophthalmic cause.

Visual fields
- Test the *temporal peripheral fields* of both open eyes by confrontation.
  - Sit opposite the patient and ask the patient to look at your nose. Bring a small object (pin or waggling finger) forwards from behind patient's ear in upper and lower lateral quadrants and ask when it can be seen.
  - If temporal fields are full there is no need to cover the other eye, but this must be done in field of binocular vision.

The patient must fully understand the test.

- Test for the *nasal peripheral fields*, with other eye covered.

  Defects in the central field (scotomata) or an enlarged blindspot can be assessed by confrontation of patient and physician and comparing their visual fields with a small red pin held in a plane midway between them. The other eye needs to be closed, and the patient asked to look at examiner's eye.

  This is a crude test and small areas of loss of vision may need to be formally tested with a perimeter or Bjerrum screen.

- Test for *sensory inattention*.
  - hold your hands between you and the patient, one opposite each ear and waggle forefingers simultaneously. Ask which moves. With a central defect, patient may not recognise movement, although fields full to formal testing.

- In a semiconscious patient a gross homonymous hemianopia can be detected by a reflex blink to your hand rapidly passing by the eye towards the ear (menace reflex).

✶ Visual
Inattention ✶

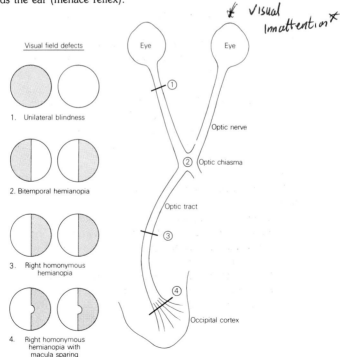

Visual field defects

1. Unilateral blindness

2. Bitemporal hemianopia

3. Right homonymous hemianopia

4. Right homonymous hemianopia with macula sparing

Eye

Eye

① Optic nerve

② Optic chiasma

Optic tract

③

④

Occipital cortex

Examine the fundi

- Start with the ophthalmoscope at + 12 dioptres (red numbers). Look at the cornea and lens. Look for the cataract (opacities on the lens) or corneal abrasions.
- Look at the retina and turn the ophthalmoscope dial until the retina comes into focus.
- Look at the disc. Check particularly for:
  - *optic atrophy* (pale disc)
  - *papilloedema* (pink; blurred edges of disc; dilated veins).
       If there is papilloedema, hypertension and raised intracranial pressure are the most common causes
  - *glaucoma* (deep cupping of whole of disc).
- Look at the arteries:
  - narrowed in hypertension with an increased light reflex.
    Hypertension grading:
    - (i) Narrow arteries.
    - (ii) Nipping of veins by arteries.
    - (iii) Haemorrhages and exudates.
    - (iv) Papilloedema.

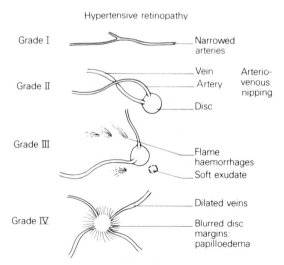

Hypertensive retinopathy

Grade I — Narrowed arteries

Grade II — Vein; Artery; Disc — Arterio-venous nipping

Grade III — Flame haemorrhages; Soft exudate

Grade IV — Dilated veins; Blurred disc margins: papilloedema

- Look at the retina for exudates, haemorrhages, choroiditis.
  - *Diabetes 'background retinopathy'*: — microaneurysms (dots)
    - deep haemorrhages (blots)
    - hard exudates (circum-scribed irregular hard, shiny white patches).
    - *soft exudates* (cotton wool spots) signify nerve swelling from local retinal infarction.
  - *'proliferative retinopathy'* — new vessels.

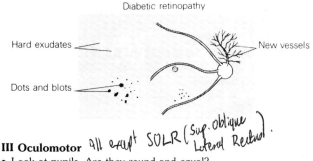

Diabetic retinopathy

Hard exudates — New vessels

Dots and blots —

III Oculomotor All exupt SOLR (Sup. oblique Lateral Rectus).

- Look at pupils. Are they round and equal?
- *Light reflex*. Shine bright light from torch into each pupil in a dimly lit room. Do pupils contract?
- *Accommodation reflex*. Ask patient to look at distant object, and then at your finger 10–15 cm from nose — do pupils contract?

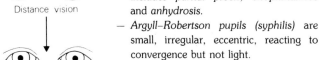

Small pupils:
  - opiates
  - *Horner's syndrome (sympathetic defect)* includes *partial ptosis, enophthalmos* and *anhydrosis.*
  - *Argyll–Robertson pupils (syphilis)* are small, irregular, eccentric, reacting to convergence but not light.

Distance vision

Sudden close vision

Large pupils:
  - alcohol
  - sympathomimetics

— *Holmes–Adie pupil:* large, slowly reacting to light.
— *cortical blindness* — no pupil response to light but good response to accommodation
— *occular blindness* — light reaction from other eye (consensual response) but not from the affected eye.

III Oculomotor

IV Trochlear

VI Abducens

External ocular movements
• Test the eye movements in the four cardinal directions using your finger at 1 metre distance. Look for abnormal eye movements and ask:
• 'Tell me if you see double'.

>   Upward gaze and convergence is often reduced in uncooperative patients.

• To detect minor lesions:
  — find direction of gaze with maximum separation of images.
  — cover one eye and ask which image has gone.

>   Peripheral image is seen by the eye that is not moving fully.

  — peripheral image displaced in direction of action of weak muscle, e.g. maximum diplopia on gaze to left. Left eye sees peripheral image which is displaced laterally. Therefore left lateral rectus is weak.

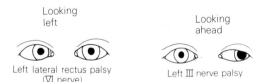

Looking left

Left lateral rectus palsy
(VI nerve)

Looking ahead

Left III nerve palsy

Diplopia may not be due to a single muscle or nerve lesion:
- paralytic strabismus (squint)
- III n. palsy: ptosis, large fixed pupil, eye can be abducted only.
- IV n. palsy: diplopia when eye looks down or inwards.
- VI n. palsy: abduction paralysed
- concomitant strabismus, e.g. childhood ocular lesion — constant angle between eyes.
- conjugate ocular palsy: supranuclear palsies affecting co-ordination rather than muscle weakness. Inability to look in particular direction.

Ptosis
Drooping of upper eyelid.
- complete — III nerve palsy
- incomplete — partial III palsy
  - muscular weakness, e.g. myasthenia gravis (from anti-acetylcholine receptor antibodies)
  - sympathetic tone decrease with *Horner's syndrome* (also small pupils — enopthalmos and decreased sweating on face)
  - partial Horner's syndrome (small irregular pupils with ptosis) in autonomic neuropathy of diabetes and syphilis.

Nystagmus
• Test with the eyes deviated to right, left and upwards. Keep object within binocular field as nystagmus often normal in extremes of gaze. Avoid hedging with 'nystagmoid jerks' — make up your mind.
- *Cerebellar* — fast movement to side of gaze (on both sides)
  - increased when look to lesion.
  e.g. from cerebellar or brainstem lesion or drugs (ethanol, phenytoin).
- *Vestibular* — fast movement only in one direction: away from lesion
  - more marked when look away from lesion.
  e.g. from inner ear, vestibular disease or brainstem lesion.

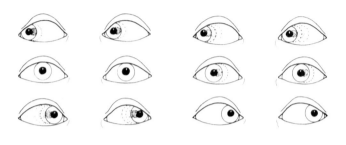

Left Cerebellar Lesion   Left Vestibular Lesion

V Trigeminal

Sensory
• Test light touch in all three divisions with cotton wool. Pinprick usually only if needed to delineate anaesthetic area.

Corneal reflex — sensory V and motor VII
• Ask the patient to look up and touch the cornea with a wisp of cotton wool. Both eyes should blink.

> The corneal reflex is easily prompted incorrectly by eliciting the 'eyelash' or 'menace' reflex.

Motor — muscles of jaw
• Ask the patient to open his mouth against resistance, and look to see if jaw descends in midline. Palsy of the nerve causes deviation of the jaw to the side of the lesion.

Fifth nerve palsies are very rare in isolation.

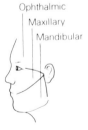

Ophthalmic
  Maxillary
    Mandibular

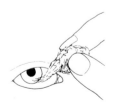

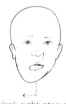

Weak right pterygoid

Jaw jerk — only if other neurological findings, e.g. upper motor neurone lesion. Increased jaw jerk is only present if there is a bilateral upper motor neurone fifth nerve lesion, e.g. bilateral strokes or pseudo bulbar palsy.

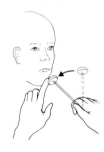

Put your forefinger gently on the patient''s loosely opened jaw. Tap your finger gently with a tendon hammer. Explain the test to the patient or relaxation of his jaw will be impossible. A brisk jerk is a positive finding.

Taste: can only be tested easily on anterior 2/3 of tongue (V chorda tympani through VII). Torch battery test quick and reliable. Dropping salt sugar, etc., on tongue not easy to interpret.

VII Facial nerve
- Ask the patient to:
    - raise his eye-brows
    - close his eyes tightly
    - show you his teeth.

Demonstrate these to the patient yourself if necessary.

Lower motor neurone lesion: all muscles on the side of the lesion are affected, e.g. *Bell's palsy.* Widened palpebral fissure, weak blink, dropped mouth.

Upper motor neurone lesion: only the lower muscles are affected, i.e. mouth drops to one side but eye-brows raise normally. This is because the upper half of the face is bilaterally innervated. This abnormality is very common in a hemiparesis.

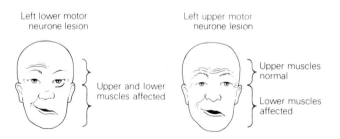

Left lower motor neurone lesion

Upper and lower muscles affected

Left upper motor neurone lesion

Upper muscles normal

Lower muscles affected

VIII Auditory

Vestibular
No easy bedside test for this nerve except looking for nystagmus.

Acoustic
• Block one ear by pressing the tragus. Whisper numbers increasingly loudly until the patient can repeat them. A ticking watch may be more useful.

More accurate tests of this nerve are as follows.

(i) *Rinnes' Test*. Place a high-pitched vibrating, tuning fork on the mastoid. When the patient says the sound stops, hold the fork at the meatus.
If still heard:
    — air conduction > bone conduction (normal or nerve deafness)
If not heard:
    — air conduction < bone conduction (middle ear conduction defect)

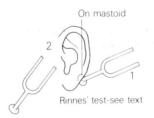

Rinnes' test-see text

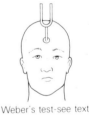

Weber's test-see text

(ii) *Weber's Test*. Hold a vibrating tuning fork in the middle of the patient's forehead. If the sound is heard to one side, middle ear deafness exists on that side or the opposing ear has nerve deafness.

IX Glossopharyngeal — Taste post ⅓ of tongue

• Ask patient to 'Ahh' and watch for symmetrical upwards movement of uvula — pulled away from weak side.
• Touch the back of the pharynx with an orange-stick or spatula gently. If the patient gags the nerve is intact.

This 'gag' reflex depends on the IX and X nerve, the former being the sensory side and the latter the motor aspect.

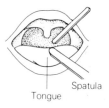

Spatula

Tongue

X Vagus

- Ask if the patient can swallow normally.

    There are so many branches of the vagus nerve that it is impossible to be sure it is all functioning normally. If the vagus is seriously damaged, swallowing is a problem; spillage into the lungs may occur.

- Dysarthria (see p. 78).

XI Accessory

- Ask the patient to flex, pressing his chin against your resisting hand. Observe if both sternomastoids contract normally.
- Ask the patient to raise both shoulders. If he cannot, the trapezius muscle is not functioning.

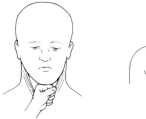
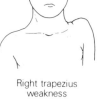

Right trapezius
weakness

Failure of the trapezius on one side is often associated with a *hemiplegia*. Traumatic cutting of the accessory nerve used to occur when tuberculous lymph glands of the neck were being excised.

XII Hypoglossal

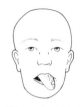

Left hypoglossal lesion

• Ask the patient to put out his tongue. If it protrudes to one side, this is the side of the weakness.

• Look for fasciculation or wasting with mouth open.

Tongue 'pushed' to weakside — deviating to left on protrusion from left hypoglossal lesion.

LIMBS AND TRUNK

General inspection

• Look at the patient's *resting and standing posture*.

Hemiplegia — flexed upper limb, extended lower limb.

Wrist drop — radial nerve palsy.

• Look for *abnormal movements*.

Tremor — Parkinson's — coarse rhythmical tremor at rest, lessens on movement.

— *Thyrotoxicosis* — fine tremor of out-stretched hands.

Chorea — Abrupt, involuntary repetitive 'semi-purposeful' movement.

Athetosis — Slow, continous writhing movement of limb.

Spasm — Exaggerated, involuntary musclar contraction.

• Look for *muscle wasting*. Check distribution.

— Symmetrical, e.g. *Duchenne muscular dystrophy*.

— Asymmetrical, e.g. *poliomyelitis*.

— Proximal, e.g. *limbgirdle muscular dystrophy*.

— Distal, e.g. *peripheral neuropathy*.

— Generalised, e.g. *motor neurone disease*.

— Localised, e.g. with *joint disease*.

• Look for *fasciculation*. This is irregular involuntary contractions of small bundles of muscle fibres, not perceived by the patient.

This is typical of denervation, e.g. motor neurone disease. It is caused by death of anterior horn cells.

ARMS

Inspection

In addition to general inspection:

• Ask the patient to hold both his arms straight out in front of him with eyes shut. Observe posture, and if arms remain stationary.

> *Hypotonic posture* — wrist flexed and fingers extended.
>
> *Drift* — gradually upwards may be *cerebellar*. Gradually downwards may be *pyramidal* weakness.

• Tap both arms downwards. They should reflexly return to their former position.

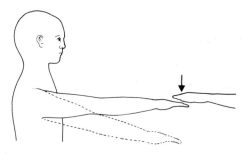

> If the arm overswings in its return to its position, weakness or *cerebellar dysfunction* may be present.

• Ask the patient to do fast finger movements: 'Play a quick tune on the piano', demonstrating this yourself. Clumsy movements can be a sensitive index of a slight *pyramidal* lesion.

Coordination

• Ask the patient to touch his nose with his index finger.

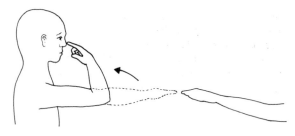

• With the patient's eyes open, ask him to touch his nose then your finger which is held up in front of him. This can be repeated rapidly with your finger moving from place to place in front of him.

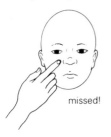

missed!

Past pointing and marked intention tremor in the absence of muscular weakness suggests *cerebellar dysfunction*. If you suspect a cerebellar abnormality check rapid alternating movements (*dysdiadochokinesis*).

— Fast rotation of the hands (*supination* and *pronation*).
— Tapping back of other hand as quickly as possible.

Tone

• Ask the patient to relax his arm and then you flex and extend his wrist or elbow. Move through a wide arc moderately slowly, at irregular intervals to prevent patient cooperation.

This is a difficult test to perform as patients often do not relax. Try to distract patient by conversation.

Hypertonia (increased tone):

— *Pyramidal:* more obvious in flexion of upper limbs, and extension of lower limbs. Occasionally 'clasp knife', i.e. alteration of tone during movement.
— *Extrapyramidal:* uniform 'lead pipe' rigidity. If associated with tremor the movement feels like a 'cog wheel'.
— *Hysterical:* increases with increased movement.

Hypotonia (decreased tone):

— Lower motor neurone lesion.
— A recent upper motor neurone lesion.
— A cerebellar lesion.
— Unconsciousness.

Muscle power

• Test power at joints against your own strength — shoulder, elbow, wrist.

Power at main joints cannot normally be overcome by permissable force.

- Compare each side. Confirm the weakness suspected by palpation of the muscle. For example:
    - 'squeeze my hands'. Present two fingers of each hand. He may hurt you if he squeezes your whole hand!
    - 'put your arms in this raised position (show him) and stop me pressing them down'.
    - 'hold my hands, and push me away'.

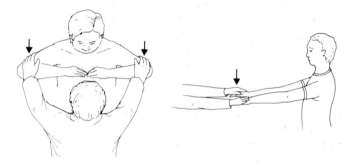

Hemiplegia: Muscles weak all down one side.

Monoplegia: Weakness of one limb.

Paraplegia: Weakness of both lower limbs.

Tetraplegia: Weakness of all four limbs.

Myasthenia: Weakness developing after repeated contractions. Most obvious in smaller muscles, e.g. repeated blinking (see ptosis, p. 87).

- If there is weakness or other neurological signs in a limb, test individual muscle groups.
    - Shoulder — abduction, extension, flexion.
    - Elbow — flexion, extension.
    - Wrist — flexion, extension: 'Hold wrists up, don't let me push them down'.
    - Finger — flexion, grasp, extension, adduction (put a piece of paper between straight fingers held in extension), abduction (with fingers in extension, ask to spread them against your face).

        0 — no active contraction.

        1 — visible as palpable contraction with no active movement.

2 — movement with gravity eliminated, i.e. in horizontal direction.

3 — movement against gravity.

4 — movement against gravity plus resistance.

5 — normal power.

Tendon reflexes

- Place arms comfortably by side with elbows flexed and hand on upper abdomen. Tell the patient to relax.
- Tap the distal end of the radius with a tendon hammer.
- Tap your forefinger or thumb over biceps tendon.
- Then hold arm across chest to tap the triceps tendon.
- Compare sides

It is essential for the patient to relax and this is not always easy, particularly in the elderly.

Increased jerks — upper motor neurone lesion (e.g. hemiparesis).

Decreased jerks — lower motor neurone lesion or acute upper motor neurone lesion.

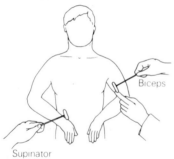

Supinator

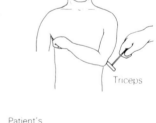

Triceps

Biceps C5–6
Supinator, triceps C7–8
Finger jerks C7–T_1

Patient's semi-flexed hand

Examiner strikes his fingers, pressing against patient's finger tips

Clonus — pressure stretching a muscle group causes rhythmical involuntary contraction. Found in marked hypertonia from stretching tendon. No need to strike tendon with tendon hammer.

TRUNK

- The superficial abdominal reflexes rarely need to be tested.
  - Lightly stroke each quadrant with an orange stick or the back of your fingernail. These are absent or decreased in an upper or lower motor neurone lesion.

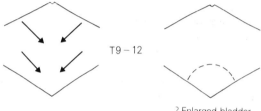

T9 – 12

? Enlarged bladder

- Cremasteric reflex T12–L1.
  - stroke inside of leg. Induces testis to rise from cremaster muscle contraction.
- Palpate the bladder
    The patient with a distended bladder will feel very uncomfortable as you palpate it.
    Many neurological lesions, sensory or motor, will lead to a distended bladder giving the patient 'retention with overflow incontinence'.
- Examine the strength of the abdominal muscles by asking the patient to attempt to sit up without using his hands.

LEGS

Inspection
- As for arms.

Coordination
• Ask the patient to run the heel of one leg up and down the shin of the other leg. Lack of coordination will be readily obvious.

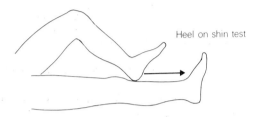

Heel on shin test

Tone
• Ask the patient to let limb go loose, lift it up and move at knee joint (hip and ankle if required).

  Difficult to assess in the legs because patients often cannot relax. Ankle clonus can be assessed at same time (see below).

Power
Hip flexion.
• Ask the patient to lift each leg in turn off bed and press down on the ankle.

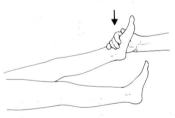

Hip extension.
• Ask patient to keep leg straight on bed, and try to lift at ankle.
• Knee: see if the patient can extend or flex his knee against your power.
• Ankle: with leg on bed, see if you can resist both dorsiflexion and plantar fexion of ankle.

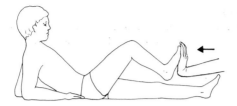

Only severe weakness will be detected because arms are weaker than legs.

Hip weakness is easily overlooked. If weakness is suspected, test the patient's ability to lift his own weight, i.e. climbing stairs, rising from a chair.

Tendon reflexes

• Test knee reflexes by passing left forearm behind both knees, supporting them partly flexed. Ask the patient to let leg go loose and tap the tendons below patella.

Compare both sides. Reflexes can be normal, brisk, (can occur in normal subjects or upper motor neurone lesion), decreased, absent, (always normal).

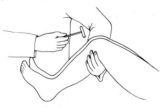

Testing the knee joint

• Test ankle reflex by flexing the knee and abducting the leg. Apply gentle pressure to the ball of the foot, with it at a right angle and tap the tendon.

Ankle jerks are often absent in the elderly.

Reinforcement — an apparently absent reflex may become present by patient pulling one hand against the other just as you strike with the hammer.

If a brisk reflex is obtained, test for *clonus*. A sharp then sustained dorsiflexion of the foot by pressure on ball of foot may result in the foot 'beating' for many seconds. Clonus confirms an increased tendon jerk and suggests an *upper motor neurone lesion*. A few symmetrical beats may be normal.

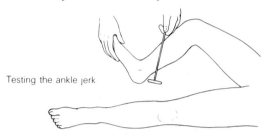

Testing the ankle jerk

Plantar reflexes

Tell patient what you are doing, and scratch the side of the sole with a firm but not painful implement (e.g. Rolls Royce car key). Watch for flexion or extension of the toes.

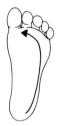

Plantar response
stimulus

Normal plantar responses–flexion of all toes. *Extensor (Babinski) response* — slow extension of the big toe with spreading of the other toes. Withdrawal from pain or tickle is rapid and not abnormal.

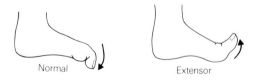

Normal   Extensor

This is often an irritating physical sign to decide if normal or abnormal. Neurologists frequently write — 'Plantar reflexes equivocal!' An extensor reflex is normal up to 6 months of age.

SENSATION

If there are no grounds to expect sensory loss, sensation can be rapidly examined.

Briefly examine each extremity. Success depends on making the patient understand what you are doing. Children are the best sensory witnesses and Dons the worst.

Vibration sense
• Test vibration sense using a 128/sec tuning fork. Place the fork on the sternum first so that the patient appreciates what vibration is. Then place the vibrating form on the lateral malleoli and wrists.

If a patient seems too good, try a non-vibrating fork or surreptitiously stop the fork vibrating and see if the patient notices. If the periphery is normal, proximal sensation need not be examined. Vibration sense is often absent in legs in the elderly patient.

Position sense — proprioception
• Show patient what you are doing.
'I am going to move your finger/toe up or down' (doing so). I want you to tell me up or down each time I move it. Now close your eyes'.
• Hold distal to joint, and side to side, with your forefinger and thumb, and make small movements in an irregular, not alternate, sequence, e.g. up, up, down, down, up, down.

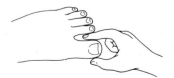

Testing position sense

Normal threshold very low — the smallest slowest passive movement you can produce in the terminal phalanges should always be correctly felt; well, nearly always. If response 'sideways' start from square one again.

Pain
• Take a pin (not a needle) and touch the sharp end of the skin. Do not draw blood. Patient's eyes can be open.
• 'Does this feel sharp like a pin prick?'

If you find sensory loss, map out that area by proceeding from abnormal to normal area of skin.

If you are uncertain about sensory loss, another but cumbersome method is to ask the patient to close his eyes, and put either the blunt or sharp end of the pin on the skin and ask which is which.

Light touch
• Eyes closed.
• 'Say 'yes'' when I touch you with a wisp of cotton wool'. Touch at irregular intervals. Compare sides of body.

Thermal sensation not examined routinely. Tests with hot and cold water in glass tubes cannot be standardised. Find an area where hot it called cold or vice versa and draw tube along skin until true temperature recognised.

2-point discrimination. Normal threshold on finger tip 2 mm. If sensory impairment peripheral or in cord, raised threshold found, e.g. 5 mm. If cortical, no threshold found.

Stereognosis tested by placing coins, keys, pen top etc. in hand and, with eyes closed, patient attempts to identify by feeling.

Sensory inattention best found with pin, not touch. Bilateral simultaneous symmetrical pinpricks are felt only on the normal side, while each is felt if applied separately. Found in cortical lesions.

GAIT

• Observe the patient as he walks in. If ataxia is suspected but not seen on ordinary walking, ask the patient to do heel-to-toe walking. (Demonstrate it yourself).

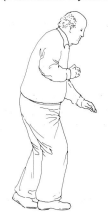

There are many examples of abnormal gait:

Parkinson's Disease. Stooped posture with most joints flexed, with small shuffling steps without swinging arms, tremor of hands.

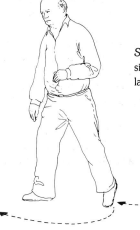

Spastic gait. Scraping toe on one or both sides as patient walks, moving foot in lateral arc to prevent this.

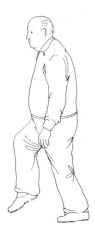

Sensory ataxia. High stepping gait, with slapping down of feet. Seen with peripheral neuropathy.

Cerebellar gait. Feet wide apart as patient walks.

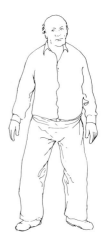

Foot drop. Toe scrapes on ground in spite of excessive lifting up leg on affected side.

Shuffling gait. Multiple little steps — typical of diffuse cerebral vascular disease.

Hysterical gait. Usually wild lurching without falling.

Romberg's test is often performed at this time but is mainly a test of position sense. Ask the patient to stand upright with his feet together and close his eyes. If there is any falling noted, the test is positive.

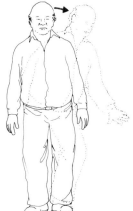

Elderly patients may fail this test and hysterics may fall sideways but stop just before they topple over. Test positive with posterier column loss of 'tabes dorsalis' of syphylis.

BACKGROUND INFORMATION

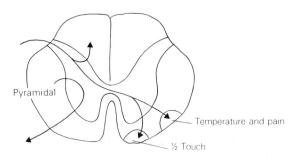

(Dorsal column) ½ Touch, position, vibration, deep pain.

Pyramidal

Temperature and pain

½ Touch

Cortical sensation. Defect shown by deficient:
— position
— tactile discrimination
— sensory inattention.

Signs of meningeal irritation:
— neck rigidity — try to flex neck. Resistance or pain?
— Kernig's sign — not as sensitive as neck rigidity.

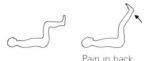

Pain in back

Straight leg raising for sciatica:
— Lift straight leg until pain in back. Then slightly lower until no pain and then dorsiflex foot to 'stretch' sciatic nerve → pain.

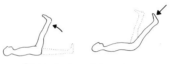

Pain in back and down leg

Summary of common signs

Lower motor neurone lesion
— wasting
— fasciculation?
— hypotonia
— power diminished
— absent reflexes
— ± sensory loss
— T_1 palsy — weak finger adduction and abduction
— radial palsy — wrist drop
— median nerve palsy — adductor policis brevis.

Upper motor neurone lesion
— no wasting
— extended arms — hand drifts down
— overswing when hands are tapped
— clumsy 'piano playing'
— hypertonia — spastic flexed upper limbs, extended lower limbs
        — clasp knife.

— power diminished
— increased tendon reflexes ($\pm$ clonus)
— absent abdominal reflexes
— extensor plantar response
— $\pm$ sphincter disturbance
— spastic gait — extended stiff leg with foot drop
             — arm does not swing, held flexed.

N.B. 'Level' first. Pathology next.

Cerebellar dysfunction

— no wasting
— hypotonia with overswing
— intention tremor
— inability to execute rapid alternating movements (dysdiadocho-kinesia)
— ataxic gait
— nystagmus
— scanning or staccato speech
— inco-ordination not improved by sight, cf. sensory defect.

Extra pyramidal dysfunction — Parkinson's disease

— flexed posture of body, neck, arms and legs
— expressionless, impassive faces, staring eyes
— 'pill rolling' tremor of hands at rest
— delay in initiating movements
— tone — lead pipe' rigidity, possibly with 'cog-wheeling'
— normal power and sensation
— speech slurred
— gait — shuffling small steps, possibly with difficulty starting or stopping.

Chapter 7
Basic Examination, Notes and Diagnostic Principles

THE BASIC EXAMINATION

In practice, one cannot attempt to elicit every single physical sign for each system. Basic signs should be sought on every examination and if there is any hint of abnormality, additional physical signs can be elicited to confirm the suspicion. Listed below are the 'basic' examinations of the systems which will enable you to complete a routine examination adequately but not excessively.

- *General examination*
  - Is the patient well or ill?
  - Look at temperature chart or take patient's temperature.
  - Any obvious abnormality?
- *General and cardiovascular system*
  - Observation — dyspnoea, distress.
  - Blood pressure.
  - Hands — temperature
    - nails e.g. clubbing
      - liver palms.
  - Pulse — rate, rhythm, character.
  - Axillae — lymph nodes.
  - Neck — lymph nodes.
  - Face and eyes — anaemia, jaundice.
  - Tongue and fauces — central cyanosis.
  - Jugular venous pulse (JVP) — height and waveform.
  - Apex beat — position and character.
  - Parasternal — heave or thrills.
  - Stethoscope — heart sounds, added sounds, murmurs
    - listen in all four areas with stethoscope diaphram
    - lie patient on left side, bell of stethoscope — MS
    - sit patient up, lean forward, breathe out — AI.
- *Respiratory system*
  - Observation.
  - Trachea — position.

— *Front of chest* — movement
                  — percuss — compare sides
                  — auscultate.
— *Back of chest* — movement
                  — percuss — particularly level of bases
                  — auscultate.
— Examine sputum.

- ***Examine spine***
- ***Abdomen***
  - Lie patient flat.
  - Feel femoral pulses and inguinal lymph nodes.
  - Herniae.
  - Look at abdomen — ask if pain or tenderness.
  - Palpate abdomen gently — generally all over? masses
                              — liver — then percuss
                              — spleen — then percuss
                              — kidneys
                              — (ascites if indicated).
  - (Auscultate if indicated).
  - Males — genitals.
  - Per rectum (PR) (only if given permission) — usually at end of examination.
  - Per vaginum (PV) — rarely by student.
- ***Legs***
  - Observation.
  - Arterial pulses
  (joints if indicated).
  - Neurology:

reflexes — knees	tone	
— ankles	power	only if indicated
— plantar responses	co-ordination	
sensation — pin prick	position	
— vibration	cottonwool	only if indicated
	temperature	

- **Arms**
  - Posture out-stretched hands, eyes closed, rapid finger movements.
  - Finger–nose co-ordination:

  reflexes — triceps   tone   } only
          — biceps   power   } if indicated
          — supinator

  sensation — pin prick   vibration
        position   } only
        cotton wool   } if indicated
        temperature

- **Cranial nerves**
  - I (if indicated).
  - II Eyes — reading print
    - pupils — torch and accommodation
    - ophthalmoscope — fundi
    - fields.
  - III IV VI Eye movements — 'Do you see double?'
    Note nystagmus.
  - V VII Open mouth
    Grit teeth — feel masseters
    Sensation — cotton wool
    (Corneal reflex — if indicated)
    (Taste — if indicated)
  - VIII Hearing — watch at each ear
    (Rinne, Weber if indicated)
  - IX X Fauces movement
  - IX Shrug shoulders
  - XII Put out tongue
- **Walk**
  - Look for gait.
- **Herniae and varicose veins.**

EXAMPLE OF NOTES

Patient's name: *Age:*   *Occupation:*
Date of admission:
Complains of:
   — List, in patient's words.
History of present illness:
   — Last well.
   — Chronological order, with both actual date of onset, and time previous to admission.
   — Detailed description of each symptom (even if appears irrelevant).
   — (May include history from informant — in which case state this is so).
   — Then detail other questions which seem relevant to possible differential diagnoses.
   — Then *functional enquiry*, 'check' system for other symptoms.
   — (Minimal statement in notes — weight, appetite, digestion, bowels, micturition, menstruation, if appropriate).

Past history:
   — Chronological order.

Family history:

Personal and social history:
   — Must include details of home circumstances, dependants, patient's occupation.
   — Effect of illness on life and its relevance to foreseeable discharge of patient.
   — Smoking. Alcohol. Medications.

Physical examination:
   — General appearance, etc.
   — Then record findings according to systems.
      Minimal statement:
      Healthy, well nourished woman.
      Afebrile, not anaemic, icteric or cyanosed.
      No enlargement of lymph nodes.

No clubbing.
Breasts and thyroid normal.

CVS: BP, pulse rate and rhythm.
JVP not raised.
Apex position.
Heart sounds 1 and 2, no murmurs.

RS: Chest and movements normal.
Percussion note normal.
Breath sounds vesicular.
No other sounds.

AS: Tongue and fauces normal.
Abdomen normal, no tenderness.
Liver, spleen, kidneys, bladder impalpable.
No masses felt.
Hernial orifices normal.
Rectal examination normal.
Vaginal examination not performed.
Testes normal.

CNS: Alert and intelligent.
Pupils equal, regular, react equally to light and accommodation.
Fundi normal.
Normal *eye* movements.
Other cranial nerves normal.
Limbs normal.

KJ	+	+
AJ	+	+
P	↓	↓

Touch and vibration normal.
Spine and joints normal.
Gait normal.

Pulses (including dorsalis pedis and posterior tibial) palpable.

Summary

Write a few sentences only:

— Salient positive features of history and examination.
— Include home circumstances.
— Include relevant negative information.

PROBLEM LIST AND DIAGNOSES

After your history and examination, make a list of:
  — the diagnoses you have been able to make
  — problems or abnormal findings which need explaining, for
     example — symptoms or signs
                 — poor social background
                 — laboratory results
                 — drug sensitivities.
It is best to separate the 'current problems' of actual or potential clinical significance requiring treatment or follow-up, from the 'inactive problems'. An example is:

Active problems	*Date*
1. Unexplained episodes of fainting	1 week
2. Angina	since 1985
3. Hypertension — blood pressure 190/100	1985
4. Chronic renal failure — plasma creatinine 200 μmol/litre	August 1989
5. Widower, unemployed, lives on own	
6. Smokes 40 cigarettes per day	
Inactive problems	
1. Thyrotoxicosis treated by partial thyroidectomy	1963
2. Hydrallazine — induced skin rash	1986

At first you will have difficulty knowing which problems to put down separately, and which can be covered under one diagnosis and a single entry. It is therefore advisable to rewrite the problem list if a problem resolves or can be explained by a diagnosis. When you have some experience, it will be appropriate to fill out the problems on a complete problem list at the front of the notes:

Active problems Include symptoms, signs, unexplained abnormal investigations, social and psychiatric problems	Date	*Inactive problems* Include major past illness, operation or hypersensitivities. Do not include problems requiring active care.	Date

From the problem list, you should be able to make:

1. **Differential diagnosis** including that which you think is most likely.
   Remember — common diseases occur commonly

   — an unusual manifestation of a common disease is more likely than an uncommon disease.

   — when you hear hoof beats, think of horses, not zebras.

   — do not necessarily be put off by some aspect which doesn't fit. (What is the farmer's friend which has four legs, wags its tail and says 'cockadoodle doo'? A dog and the sound was from another animal).

2. **Possible diagnostic investigations** you feel are appropriate.

3. **Management and therapy** you think are appropriate.

4. **Prognostic implications**.

Diagnoses

The diagnostic terms which physicians use often relate to different levels of understanding:

Disordered function	imobile painful joint ↑	breathlessness ↑	angina ↑
Structural lesion	osteoarthritis ↑	anaemia ↑	narrow coronary artery ↑
Pathology	iron deposition fibrosis ↑	iron deficiency ↑	aortitis ↑
Aetiology	inherited disorder of iron metabolism (haemo-chromatosis)	bleeding duodenal ulcer	*Treponema pallidum* (syphilis)

Different problems require diagnoses at different levels, which may change as further information becomes available. Thus, a patient on admission may be diagnosed as '*pyrexia of unknown origin*'. After plain X-ray abdomen, he may be found to have a '*renal mass*' which on a

CAT Scan becomes '*perinephric abscess*', which from blood cultures is found to be '*Staphylococcus aureus*' infection. For a complete diagnosis all aspects should be known, but often this is not possible.

Note many terms are used as a diagnosis but, in fact, cover considerable ignorance, e.g. *diabetes mellitus* (originally sweet-tasting urine', but now diagnosed also by high plasma glucose) is not more than a descriptive term of disordered function, and *sarcoid* relates to a pattern of symptoms and a pathology of 'noncaseating granulomata' of which the aetiology is unknown.

Progress notes

While the patient is in hospital, full progress notes should be kept
— to give a complete picture of how the diagnosis was established
— how the patient was treated
— the evolution of the illness
— any complications that occurred.

These notes are as important as the account of the original examination. In acute cases record daily changes in signs and symptoms. In chronic cases, the relevant systems should be re-examined at least once a week and the findings recorded.

Is is useful to separate different aspects of the illness:
— symptoms
— signs
— laboratory investigations.
— general assessment, e.g. apparent response to therapy
— further plan, which would include educating the patient and his family about the illness.

Objective findings such as alterations in weight, improvement in colour, pulse, character of respirations or fluid intake and output are more valuable than purely *subjective statements* such as 'feeling better' or 'slept well'.

When appropriate, daily blood pressure readings or analyses of the urine should be recorded.

An account of all ward procedures such as aspirations of chest should be included.   Specifically record:
— the findings and comments of the physician or surgeon in charge
— results of a case conference
— an opinion from another department.

Dr Larry Weed proposed a system of notekeeping in which the history — examination constituted a 'Data Base'. All subsequent notes are structured according to the *specific numbered problems* in a 'Problem List'. Problem oriented records really require a special system of note keeping. The full system is therefore not often used, but the problem list is an extremely valuable check that all aspects of his illness are being covered.

Serial investigations

The results of these should be collected together in a *table* on a special sheet. When any large series of investigations is made, e.g. serial blood counts, erythrocyte sedimentation rates or multiple biochemical analyses, the results can also be expressed by a *graph*.

Operation notes

In patients undergoing surgical treatment, an operation note must be written immediately after the operation. Do not trust your memory for any length of time as several similar problems may be operated on at the one session. Even if you are distracted by an emergency, the notes must be written up the same day as the operation. These notes should contain definite statements on the following facts:

* Name of surgeon performing the operation and his assistant.
* Name of anaesthetist and anaesthetic used.
* Type and dimension of incision used.
* Pathological condition found, and mention of anatomical variations.
* Operative procedures carried out.
* Method of repair of wound and suture materials used.
* Whether drainage used, material used, and whether sutured to wound.
* Type of dressing used.

Post-operative notes

Within the first 2 days after operation note:
  — the general condition of the patient
  — any complication or troublesome symptom, e.g. pain, haemorrhage, vomiting, distension, etc.
  — any treatment.

Discharge note

A full statement of the patient's condition on discharge should be written:

— final diagnosis
— active problems
— medication and other therapies
— plan
— what the patient has been told
— where the patient has gone, and what help is available
— when the patient is next being seen
— an estimate of the prognosis.

If the patient dies, the student must attend the post mortem and then complete his note by a short account of the autopsy findings.

Chapter 8
Assessment of Disability Including Care of the Elderly

It is important, particularly in the elderly, to assess whether the patient has disability:
— which interferes with normal life and aspirations
— makes the patient dependent on others — requires temporary assistance for specific problems
— occasional or regular assistance long-term
— supervised accommodation
— nursing home with 24-hour care.

It is necessary to assess the following in a patient.
— Ability to do day-to-day functions.
— Mental ability including confusion or dementia.
— Emotional state and drive.

The descriptive terms used for disability have specific definitions in a World Health Organization classification.
— *Impairment* — any loss or abnormality of anatomical, physiological or psychological function, *i.e. systems or parts of body that do not work*.
— *Disability* — any restrictions or lack of ability (due to an impairment) to perform an activity within the range considered normal, *i.e. activities that cannot be done*.
— *Handicap* — a limitation of normal occupation because of impairment or disability, *i.e. social consequences*.

Thus: — a hemiparesis is an impairment
— an inability to wash or dress is a disability
— an inability to do an occupation is a handicap.

The introductory clinical training in the first few chapters concentrates on evaluation of impairments. Disability and handicap are not always given due attention and are the practical and social aspects of the disease process. It is a mistake if the doctor is preoccupied by impairments, since the patient often perceives disability as the major problem.

The impairments, disability and handicap should have been covered in a normal history and examination, but it can be helpful to bring together important facts to provide an overall assessment.

A summary description of a patient may include the following.

— *Aetiology* — familial hypercholesterolaemia.
— *Pathology* — atheroma
             — right middle cerebral artery thrombosis.
— *Impairment* — left hemiparesis
             — paralysed left arm, fixed in flexion
             — upper motor neurone signs in left arm and face.
— *Disability* — difficulty during feeding. Cannot drive his car.
— *Handicap* — can no longer work as a travelling salesman
             — embarrassed to socialise.
— *Social circumstances* — wife can cope with day-to-day living, but lack of income from his occupation and withdrawal from society present major problems.

ASSESSMENT OF IMPAIRMENT

The routine history and examination will often reveal impairments. Additional standard clinical measures are often used to assist quantitation, e.g. — treadmill exercise test
        — peak flow meter
        — MRC scale of muscle power
        — making five-pointed star from matches (to detect dyspraxia in hepatic encephalopathy)

Questionnaires can similarly provide a semi–quantitative index of important aspects of impairment and give a brief short–hand description of a patient. The role of the questionnaire is in part a check list to make sure the key questions are asked.

Cognitive function

In the elderly impaired cognitive function can be assessed by a standard *Mental Test Score* introduced by Hodkinson. The test assumes normal communication skills. One mark each is given for correct answers to 10 standard questions.

— Age of patient.
— Time (to nearest hour).
— Address given, for recall at end of test, e.g. 42 West Street or 92 Columbia Road.
— Name of hospital or area of town if at home.
— Year (if January of February the previous year is accepted).
— Date of birth of patient.
— Month.
— Years of first world war.
— Name of monarch in UK, president in USA.
— Count backwards from 20 to 1 (no errors allowed unless self corrected).
— [Check recall of address.]

This scale is a basic test of gross defects of memory and orientation and is designed to detect cognitive impairment. It has the advantages of brevity, relative lack of culture–specific knowledge and widespread use. In the elderly, 8–10 is normal, 7 is probably normal, 6 or less is abnormal.

Specific problems, such as confusion or wandering at night are not included in the mental test score, and indicate that the score is a useful check list but is not a substitute for a clinical assessment.

Affect and drive

Motivation and depression are important determinants of successful rehabilitation.

ASSESSMENT OF DISABILITY

Assessing patients disabilities is often the key to successful management.
Make a list of disabilities separate from other problems e.g. diagnoses, symptoms, impairments, social problems.

This list can assist with setting priorities, including which investigations or therapies are most likely to be of benefit to the patient.

Activities of daily living (ADL)

These are key functions, which in the elderly affect the degree of independence. Several scales of disability have been used. One of these, the *Barthel index of ADL* records the following disabilities that can affect self-care and mobility.

— Continence, urinary and faecal.
— Ability to use toilet.
— Grooming.
— Feeding.
— Dressing.
— Bathing.
— Transfer, e.g. chair to bed.
— Walking.
— Using stairs.

The assessment denotes the current state and not the underlying cause or the potential improvement. It does not include cognitive functions or emotional state. It emphasises independence, so a catheterised patient who can competently manage the device achieves the full score for urinary incontinence. The total score provides an overall estimate or summary of dependence, but between patient comparisons are difficult as they may have different combinations of disability. As a rough guide, a score of 14 indicates disability which is usually compatible with the level of support in a residential home, whereas a score of 10 requires maximum support and a carer in attendance.

Instrumental activities of daily living (IADL)

These are slightly more complex activities relating to an individual's ability to live independently. They often require special assessment in the home environment.

— Preparing a meal.
— Doing light housework.
— Using transport.
— Managing money.
— Shopping.
— Doing laundry.
— Taking medications.
— Using a telephone.

Communication

In the elderly, difficulty in communication is a frequent problem, and impairment of the following may need special attention.
- Deafness (do the ears need syringing? Is a hearing aid required?).
- Speech (is dysarthria due to lack of teeth?).
- An alarm to call for help when required.
- Aids for reading, e.g. spectacles, magnifying glass.
- Resiting or adaption of doorbell, telephone, radio or television.

ANALYSING DISABILITIES AND SETTING OBJECTIVES

After writing a list of disabilities, it is necessary to make a possible treatment plan with specific objectives. The plan needs to be realistic. A multidisciplinary, team approach, including social workers, physiotherapists, occupational therapists, nurses and doctors in usually essential in rehabilitation of elderly patients.

The overall aims in treating the elderly include the following.
- To make diagnoses if feasible, particularly of treatable illnesses.
- To comfort and alleviate problems and stresses even if one cannot cure.
- To add life to years even if cannot add years to life.

Specific aspects which may need attention include the following.
- Alleviate social problems if feasible.
- Improve heating, clothing, toilet facilities, cooking facilities.
- Arrange support services, e.g. help with shopping, provision of meals, attendance to day centre.
- Regular visits from nurse or other helper.
- Make sure family, neighbours and friends understand the situation.
- Help with sorting out finances.
- Provide aids, e.g. — large handled implements
  - walking frame or stick
  - slip–on shoes
  - handles by bath or toilet.
- Help to keep as mobile as feasible.

— Facilitate visits to hearing–aid centre, optician, chiropodist, dentist.
— Ensure medications are kept to a minimum, and the instructions and packaging are suitable.

CAUSES OF DISABILITIES

Specific disabilities may have specific causes which can be alleviated. In the elderly common problems include the following.

— Confusion — darkness
             — deafness
             — infection
             — side effects of drugs
             — other precipitating illnesses, e.g. heart failure, respiratory failure.
— Incontinence — WC far away, e.g. upstairs
             — physical restriction of gait
             — urine infection
             — faecal impaction
             — uterine prolapse
             — diabetes.
— 'Off legs' — neurological impairment
             — unsuspected fracture of leg
             — depressed
             — general illness, e.g. infection, heart failure, renal failure, hypothermia, hypothyroid, diabetes, hypokalaemia.
— Falls — insecure carpet
             — dark stairs
             — poor vision, e.g. cataracts
             — postural hypotension
             — cardiac arrhythmias
             — epilepsy
             — neurological deficit, e.g. Parkinson's disease, hemiparesis
             — cough or micturition syncope
             — intoxication.

Chapter 9
Communicating

PRESENTATIONS TO DOCTORS

Medicine is a subject in which you have to be able to talk. The more practice you get, the better you will become and the more confident you will appear in front of doctors, nurses and patients. 'Confidence' displayed by the doctor is an important aspect of therapy and the value to the patient of a doctor who can speak lucidly is enormous.

Practice talking to yourself in a mirror avoiding any breaks or interpolating the word 'er'. Open a textbook, find a subject and give a little talk on it to yourself. Even if you do not know anything about the subject you will be able to make up a few coherent sentences once you are practised.

A presentation is not the time to demonstrate you have been thorough and have asked all questions, but is a time to show you can intelligently assemble the essential facts.

In all presentations, give the salient positive findings, and the relevant negative findings. For example:
- in a patient with progressive dyspnoea, state if patient has ever smoked.
- a patient with icterus, state if patient had not been abroad, has not had any recent injections or drugs, or contact with other jaundiced patients.

Three presentations are likely to be encountered:

Presentation of a case to a meeting
This must be properly prepared, including visual aids as necessary. The principal details, shown on an overhead projector, are helpful as a reminder to you, and the audience may more easily remember the details of a case if they 'see' as well as 'hear' them.

- Practice your presentation from beginning to end and leave nothing to chance.
- Do not speak to the screen; speak to the audience.
- Do not crack jokes, unless you are confident that they are apposite.
- Do not make sweeping statements.
- Remember what you are advised to do in a court of law — dress up, stand up, speak up, shut up.
- Read up about the disease or problem before hand so that you can answer any queries.
- Read a recent leading article, review or research publication on the subject

In many hospitals it is expected that you present an apposite, original article. Be prepared to evaluate and criticise the manuscript. If your seniors cannot give you references, look up the subject in *Index Medicus*, or large textbooks, or ask the always helpful librarian for advice. Laboriously repeating standard information from a textbook is often a turn-off. A recent series or research paper is more educational for you, and more interesting for the audience.

The *presentation overhead* summarises any presentation:

Mr A.B.   Age: x years   Brief description e.g. occupation

Complains of:
State in patient's words — for x period.

History of present complaint:
- essential details
- other relevant information, e.g. risk factors
- relevant negative information relating to possible diagnoses
- extent to which symptoms or disease limit normal activity
- other symptoms — mention briefly.

Past history:
- briefly inactive problems
- information about active problems, or inactive problems relevant to present illness
- record allergies including type of reaction to drugs.

Family history:
— brief information about parents, otherwise detail only if relevant.

Social history:
— brief unless relevant
— give family social background
— occupation and previous occupations
— any other special problems
— tobacco or ethanol abuse, past or present.

Treatment:
— note all drugs with doses.

On examination:
General description
— introductory descriptive sentence, e.g. well, obese man.
— clinical signs relevant to disease
— relevant negative findings.
  Remember these findings should be descriptive data rather than your interpretation.

Problem list

Differential diagnoses:
— put in order of likelihood.

Investigations:
— relevant positive findings
— relevant negative findings
— tables or graphs for repetitive data
— photocopy an ECG or temperature chart for overhead presentation.

Progress report

Plan

Subjects which often are discussed after your presentation are:

— other differential diagnoses
— other features of presumed diagnosis that might have been present or require investigation
— pathophysiological mechanisms
— mechanisms of action of drugs and possible side effects.

After clinical discussion, be prepared to present a publication with essential details on an overhead.

Presentation of a new case on a ward round

• Good written notes are a great assistance. Do not read your notes word for word; use your notes as a reference.
• Either highlight, underline or asterisk key features you will wish to refer to, or write up a separate note-card for reference.
• Talk formally and avoid speaking too quickly or too slowly. Speak to the whole assembled group rather than a tête à tête with the consultant.
• Stand upright — it helps to make you appear confident.
• If you are interrupted by a discussion, note where you are and be ready to resume, repeating the last sentence before proceeding.

History:
The format will be similar to that on an overhead, with emphasis on positive findings and relevant negative information. A full description of the initial, main symptom is usually required.

Examination:
Once your history is complete the consultant may ask for the relevant clinical signs only. Still add in relevant negative signs you think are important.

Summary:
Be prepared to give a problem list and differential diagnoses.

If you are presenting the patient at the bedside, ensure the patient is comfortable. If the patient wishes to make an additional point or clarification, it is best to welcome this. If it is relevant it can be helpful. If irrelevant, politely say to the patient you will come back to him in a moment, after you have presented the findings. Do not appear to argue with the patient.

Brief follow-up presentations

Give a brief, orientating introduction to provide a framework on which other information can be placed. For example:

A xx year old man who was admitted xx days ago.

Long-standing problems include xxxxx (list briefly).

Presented with xx symptoms for x period.

On examination had xx signs.

Initial diagnosis of xx was confirmed/supported by/not supported by xx investigations.

He was treated by xx.

Since then xx progress

— symptoms

— examination

Start with general description and temperature chart and, if relevant, investigations.

If there are multiple active problems, describe each separately, e.g.

— firstly in regard to the xxxx.

— secondly in regard to the xxxx.

The outstanding problems are xxxx.

The plan is xxxx.

PEOPLE — INCLUDING PATIENTS

A significant number of disasters, a great deal of irritation and a lot of unpleasantness could be avoided in hospitals by proper communication. The doctor is not the 'boss' but is part of a team, all of whom significantly help the patient. You must be able to communicate properly with the nursing staff, physiotherapists, occupational therapists, administrators, ancillary staff and above all, patients.

When you first arrive on the wards it is a good idea to go and see the ward sister, physiotherapist, etc., and find out what their job is, what their difficulties are and how they view the patient, other groups, and most importantly, yourself.

Remember these points.

• **Time** — when you talk to anyone, try not to appear in a rush or they will lose concentration and not listen. A little time taken to talk to somebody properly will help enormously.

• **Listen** — active listening to someone is not easy but is essential for good communication. Many people stop talking but not all appear to be listening. Sitting down with the patient is advantageous, both in helping you to concentrate and in transmitting to the patient that you are willing to listen.

• *Smile* — grumpiness or irritation is the best way to stop a patient talking. A smile will often encourage a patient to tell you problems he would not normally do. It helps everybody to relax.

• *Reassurance* — if you appear confident and relaxed this helps others to feel the same. Being calm without excessive body movements can help. Note how a good consultant has a reassuring word for patients and allows others in the team to feel they are (or are capable of) working effectively. As a student you are not in a position to do this, but you can contribute by playing your role efficiently and calmly.

• *Humility* — no one, in particular the patient, is inferior to you.

Chapter 10
Clinical Investigations

This brief introduction to major clinical investigations starts with a general description of the major techniques, and is followed by specialised investigations in cardiology (see p. 140), respiratory medicine (see p. 145), gastroenterology (see p. 150) renal medicine (see p. 152), and neurology (see p. 154).

ULTRASOUND EXAMINATIONS

A probe which produces ultrasound (2–6 MHz) is placed on the skin, and receives reflections back from tissue, particularly inferfaces, e.g. fluid/solid, gas/fluid, gas/solid, etc.

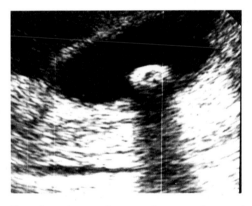

Part of an ultrasound picture showing reflections from gallstone in a gall bladder (with corresponding shadow beyond the gallstone).

Reflections are detected along a line or plane and can be shown as a two-dimensional triangular section of the underlying tissues. The scans provided as permanent records are only some of the many observations made.

The technique has the advantage of being safe, repeatable, painless non-radioactive and simple, but requires an experienced observer.

It is useful in many situations:
- organs of abdomen, including their size
  - liver — tumour, abscess, dilated bile ducts
  - gallbladder — gallstones including non-radio-opaque stones
  - pancreas — tumour, stones
  - kidneys — hydronephrosis from obstruction of ureters or pelviureteric junction
  - ovaries — cysts, tumours
  - uterus — masses, foetus in obstetrics
  - aorta — aneurysm
  - appendix — inflammatory mass or abscess
  - bowel — dilation, tumours, inflammatory masses
- thyroid — whether lumps are cystic or solid
- heart (see echocardiography, p. 141)
- blood vessels.

ENDOSCOPY

Internal organs are directly visualised, usually with a flexible fibreoptic endoscope.

Gastroscopy
A flexible 'scope is inserted by mouth after i.v. diazepam. To investigate:
- *dysphagia* — oesophageal tumour or stricture;
- *haematemesis* or *melaena* — oesophageal varices, gastric and duodenal ulcers, superficial gastric erosions, gastric carcinoma:
- *epigastric pain* — peptic ulcer, oesophagitis, gastritis, duodenitis,
- unexplained weight loss — gastric carcinoma. (See p. 150 for ERCP.)

Proctoscopy

With the patient lying in a left-lateral position on one side, with knees and hips flexed, a short tube is introduced through the anus with a removable obturator lubricated with a gel. To investigate:

— *rectal bleeding* — haemorrhoids or anal carcinoma.

Sigmoidoscopy

With the patient in left-lateral position, either a rigid tube with a removable obturator, or a flexible fibre optic endoscope is introduced. Bowel is kept patent with air from a hand pump. To investigate:

— bleeding, diarrhoea or constipation — diagnosis of *ulcerative colitis*, other *inflammatory bowel disease* or *carcinoma*. Inflammed area or lumps can be biopsied.

Colonoscopy

After the bowel is emptied with an oral purgative and a washout if necessary, the whole of the colon and possibly the terminal ileum can be examined. To investigate:

— *inflammatory bowel disease, polyps or carcinoma.*

Bronchoscopy

After i.v. diazepam, the major bronchi are observed. To investigate:

— haemoptysis or suspected bronchial obstruction, — diagnosis of *bronchial carcinoma* and for clearing *obstructed bronchi*, e.g. peanuts, plug of mucus.

Laparoscopy

After general anaesthetic, organs can be observed through a small abdominal incision, aspirated for cells or organisms, or biopsied. Sterilisation can be performed using this technique. Ova can be collected for *in vitro* fertilisation.

Cystoscopy

After local anaesthetic, a cystoscope is inserted in to the urethral meatus. To investigate:

— urinary bleeding or poor flow — diagnosis of *bladder and prostatic tumours*. Under direct vision, catheters can be inserted into ureters for *retrograde pyelogram*.

Colposcopy

Examination of cervix, usually to take a cervical smear. To investigate:
— pre-malignant changes or cancer.

NEEDLE BIOPSY

A small core of tissue (30 mm × 1 mm) is obtained through needle puncture of organs for histological diagnosis. To investigate:
— liver — *cirrhosis, alcoholic liver disease, chronic active hepatitis;*
— kidney — *glomerulonephritis, interstitial nephritis;*
— lung — usually a 'drill biopsy' using a powered rotating drill to insert a needle — *fibrosis, tumours, tuberculosis.*

Fine needle aspiration

A technique to obtain cells for diagnosis of tumours or for bacteriological diagnosis. The needle position is guided by ultrasound, CT scan or magnetic resonance imaging scan. For investigation of many unexplained lumps, e.g. pancreas, breast lumps to diagnose carcinoma.

RADIOLOGY

Conventional X-rays visualise only four basic radiographic densities: air, metal, fat, water. Air densities are black; metal densities (the most common of which are calcium and barium) are white with well defined edges; fat and water densities are grey/white.

There can be difficulty in visualising a three-dimensional structure from a two-dimensional film. One helpful rule in deciding where a lesion is situated is to note which, if any, adjacent normal landmarks are obliterated. For example, a water density lesion which obliterates the right border of the heart must lie in the right-middle lobe and not the lower lobe. A different view, e.g. lateral chest X-ray, is needed to be certain of the position of densities.

Chest X-ray

Use a systematic approach.
• PA or AP. The correct name for the usual chest study is 'a PA chest

radiograph'. This means that the anteriorly situated heart is as close to the film as possible and its image will be minimally enlarged.

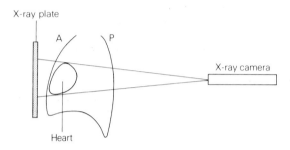

A normal 'PA' X-ray.

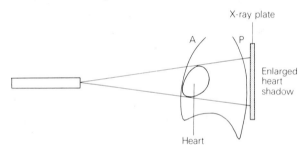

AP Chest X-ray (Portable X-ray for chest radiographs of patients in bed).

• Check sex and nationality from name on film and try to estimate age (neonate, child, middle aged, elderly).
• Measure diameter of the heart at its widest point and express it as a ratio of the diameter of the chest at its widest point. This is less than 0.5 in adults.
• Is heart shadow normal?
• Is mediastinum normal?
• Are hilar shadows normal?
• Lung fields: are markings normal? The horizontal fissure is not always visible but look for it and check its position. Look at the

pulmonary vessels. Is there upper lobe diversion, congestion, peripheral cut off? Lung shadows should be of equal intensity.
- Make sure there is no pneumothorax.
- Look at diaphragms — right normally higher than left.
- Soft tissues
- Bones: fractures, lytic or sclerotic lesions, bone density ↑ or ↓.

Abdominal radiography

This is less satisfactory than chest radiography because there are fewer contrasting densities. Air in the gut is helpful, as are the psoas lines. Try to find as many organ outlines as possible:
- Kidneys.
  - The outline of the kidneys may be seen lateral and parallel to the psoas lines, approximately opposite L1, 2 and 3. The average kidney varies between 2½ and 3½ vertebral heights.
- Liver and spleen.
  - Usually identified. Check if enlarged.
- Stomach.
  - Air filled.
- Gut.
  - Small bowel may contain air but the more obvious haustral pattern is seen in the large bowel.
- Always check for abdominal calcification and for bone or joint abnormalities.

Computerised axial tomography (CAT scan or CT scan)

A segment of the body is X-rayed at numerous angles as the apparatus rotates through 360°. A computer summarises the data from multiple pictures to provide a composite picture.
  - For organs and masses in abdomen and thorax.
  - To diagnose tumours, strokes and bleeds in major cerebral hemispheres.
  - Posterior fossa lesions less easy to visualise because of bony base of skull.
  - Disc prolapse and neoplasm in spinal cord can be visualised, but adjacent bones interfere.

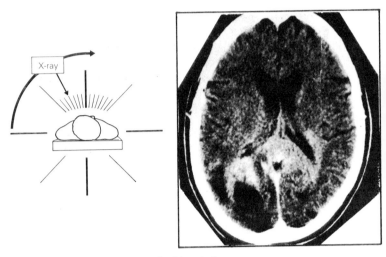

CT scan across cerebral hemispheres

Arteriography and venography

An X-ray film is taken after a radio-opaque contrast has been injected into a blood vessel.

— coronary arteriography, e.g. *coronary artery disease*;
— cerebral angiography, e.g. *aneurysm after subarachnoid haemorrhage*;

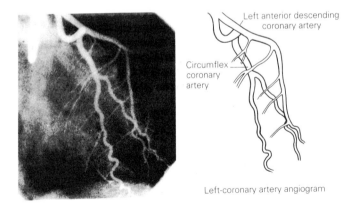

Left anterior descending coronary artery

Circumflex coronary artery

Left-coronary artery angiogram

— carotid angiography e.g. *stenoses*.
— pulmonary angiography, e.g. *pulmonary embolus* or *fistula*;
— renal angiography, e.g. *renal artery stenosis, renal tumour, phaeochromocytoma*;
— aortography and ilio-femoral angiography, e.g. *aortic aneurysm, ilio-femoral artery atheroma*;
— leg venogram, e.g. *deep venous thrombosis.*

Concurrent venous blood sampling may help localise an endocrine tumour, e.g. parathormone from an occult parathyroid tumour, catecholamines from a phaeochromocytoma, or to confirm the significance of renal artery stenosis using renal vein renin analyses.

Background subtraction angiography

Contrast is inserted rapidly via a peripheral vein or into the vessel. As the contrast passes along the artery concerned, X-ray pictures are taken.

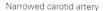
Narrowed carotid artery

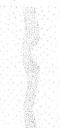

Before subtraction   After subtraction

Digital subtraction; a computer subtracts the background field leaving a clear view of the artery.

Overlay subtraction; the positive of a background film is laid over the angiogram cancelling out non-contrast features.
— Used to observe arterial stenoses or aneurysms.
— can be used to assess left-ventricular function.

Radionucleotide studies

Radioactive material can be used to study many organs, e.g. the brain, liver, spleen, heart, kidney, thyroid, lung or bone.

Technetium-99 is the most common radionucleotide used and is linked to the appropriate chemical compound or protein, e.g. monoclonal antibody, depending on the organ to be studied. Thallium-201 is used for myocardial studies.

Lesions present either as photon-abundant areas (as in bone or brain) or photon-deficient areas (as in liver, lung, hearts, etc).

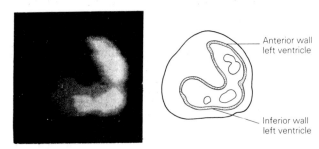

Thallium-201 study of the heart

MAGNETIC RESONANCE IMAGING

Also known as nuclear magnetic resonance (NMR).

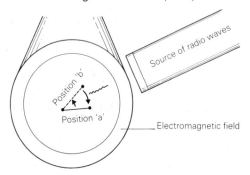

The principles of nuclear magnetic resonance

The axes of individual hydrogen ions usually lie at random but can be lined up at a particular angle by a strong magnetic field (position 'a').

When subjected to radiowaves the angle is changed (position 'b').
When the radiowaves cease position 'a' is restored by the continuing
magnetic field and a radiowave is emitted and detected.

Hydrogen MRI — the various organs of the body contain different
concentrations of hydrogen ions and so organs can be clearly seen.

Excellent for demonstrating tumours, multiple areas of demyelination of white matter in multiple sclerosis, spinal cord lesions
including disc prolapse.

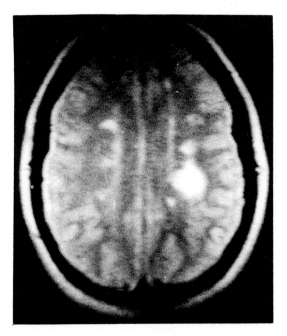

MRI scan of the brain; a hydrogen scan. The white areas are
patches of demyelination in multiple sclerosis.

Phosphorus MRI — phosphorus ions can be detected in tissue as
ATP, ADP or creatine phosphate providing *in vivo* measurement of the
energy levels of tissue for research purposes or for assessing the viability
of pre-transplanted organs.

CARDIOLOGICAL INVESTIGATIONS

Electrocardiograph (ECG) *see* p. 159.

Exercise test
Primarily for diagnosis and prognosis of angina.
— Walk on a treadmill
— Every 3 minutes speed and slope increased from approximately 1:10 at 1 mph to 1:5 at 5 mph.
— Patient stops when develops typical symptoms, *e.g.* pain.
— Test is stopped if ECG changes rapidly (ST segment depressed), arrhythmia appear, or the BP drops suddenly.
  Decreased ST segments in a specific region indicates ischaemia. This may indicate the need for medical treatment or coronary angiography.

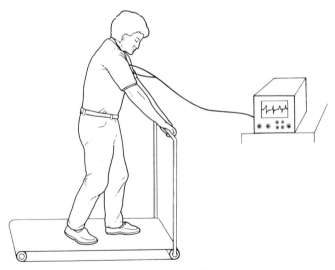

The treadmill exercise

Echocardiography

Visualises structures and function of the heart. Uses ultrasound (2–6 MHz) to reflect from interfaces in the heart, e.g. ventricle and atrial walls, heart, valves, major vessels.

M mode (single 'plane') echocardiography uses a narrow beam, and movements of the heart in that beam are visualised on moving sensitised paper.

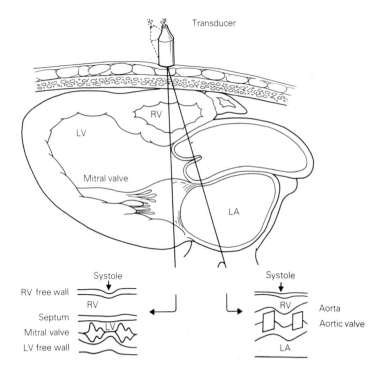

Two-dimensional (2D) echocardiography uses a scanning beam of 45° or 60° to visualise the anatomy of the heart.

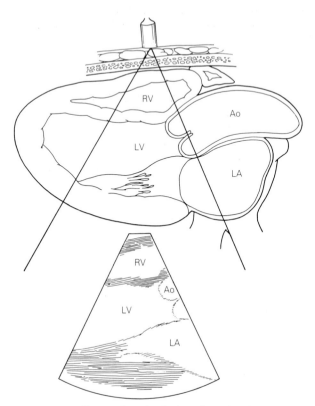

The two-dimensional echocardiograph

Echocardiography is excellent for:
— *congenital heart disease*
— *mitral stenosis* (but not other valve lesions)
— *pericardial effusion*
— *left ventricular function*, e.g. poor contraction, low ejection fraction, akinetic segment, paradoxical motion in aneurysm.

Twenty-four hour ECG tape recording

ECG worn for 24 hours (or 48 hours) and obtains on tape a continuous ECG recording during normal activities.

For diagnosis of:
- — palpitations
- — dizzy spells
- — light headedness or blackouts of possible cardiac origin.

May show episodes of:
- — atrial asystole
- — atrial or ventricular tachycardias
- — complete heart block
- — ST segment changes during angina or silent ischaemia.

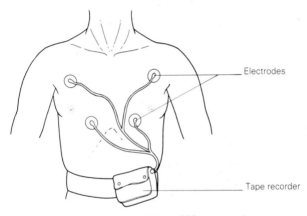

Electrodes

Tape recorder

The arrangement for the 24-hour ECG tape recorder

Cardiac catherization

With mild sedation under operating theatre conditions, thin catheters are introduced, usually via femoral artery or vein, and manipulated to the various chambers in the right and left sides of the heart.

The technique shows pressure differences (gradient) across the valve.

Contrast can be pumped rapidly into a chamber, e.g. left ventricle, and its size, shape and function can be determined (ventriculography) by X-ray pictures.

Oxygen saturations localise the presence of shunts (ASD, VSD, PDA).

In coronary arteries, injection of radio-opaque dye shows the presence and degree of atheroma (coronary angiography).

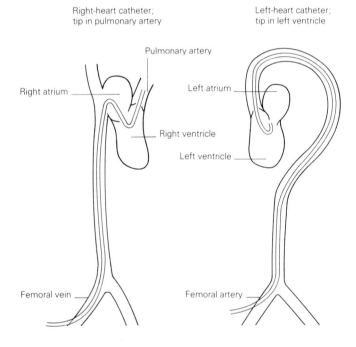

Cardiac isotopic scans

Following an injection of an isotope, pictures of the heart are taken with a gamma camera.

Thallium-209 — taken up by viable myocardium but not ischaemic myocardium, i.e. cold spot = ischaemia.

Technitium-99 labelled pyrophosphate — attached to red cells demonstrates left ventricular function by taking video pictures of the passage of blood through the heart.

RESPIRATORY INVESTIGATIONS

pH and arterial blood gases
Normal ranges
  — pH 7.35–7.45
  — P_{CO_2} 4.5–6.2 pKa
  — P_{O_2} > 10.6 pKa
  — HCO_3^- 22–26 mmol/litre.
Base excess is the amount of acid required to titrate pH to 7.4.
In ventilatory failure:
  — P_{O_2} low
  — P_{CO_2} high.
In respiratory failure from lung disease often:
  — P_{O_2} low
  — normal P_{CO_2} due to high CO_2 solubility and efficient transfer in
    lungs.
      For example, in asthma, raised CO_2 signifies tiredness and
      decreased ventilation from reduced muscular effort.

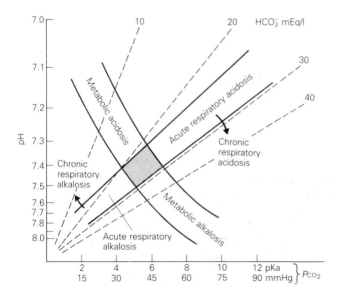

Respiratory acidosis

CO_2 retention from:
— respiratory disease with right to left shunt
— ventilatory failure — neuromuscular disease
— physical causes, e.g. flail chest, kyphoscoliosis.

Raised CO_2 leads to increased bicarbonate:

$$CO_2 + H_2O \rightleftharpoons H_2CO_3 \rightleftharpoons H^+ + HCO_3^-.$$

In chronic respiratory failure, renal compensation by excretion of H^+ and retention of HCO_3^- leads to further increased HCO_3^-, i.e. maintenance of normal pH with compensatory metabolic alkalosis.

Respiratory alkalosis

CO_2 blown off by hyperventilation — hysteria
— brainstem stimulation (rare).

— P_{O_2} normal.
— P_{CO_2} low.

If chronic, compensated by metabolic acidosis with renal retention of H^+ and excretion of HCO_3^-.

Metabolic acidosis

Excess H^+ in blood:
— ketosis — 3 OH butyric acid accumulation in diabetes or starvation;
— uraemia — lack of renal H^+ excretion;
— renal tubular acidosis: lack of H^+ or NH_4^+ excretion;
— acid ingestion — aspirin;
— lactic acid accumulation — shock, hypoxia, exercise, biguanide;
— formic acid accumulation — methanol intake;
— loss of base — diarrhoea.

Usually compensatory respiratory alkalosis, e.g. Kussmaul respiration of diabetic coma, (hyerventilation with deep breathing).

— P_{O_2} normal
— P_{CO_2} low
— To assist diagnosis, measure anion gap.

$$[Na^+] + [K^+] - [Cl^-] - [HCO_3^-] = 7\text{--}16 \text{ mmol/litre}$$

If > 16, unestimated anions are present, e.g. 3 OH butyrate, lactate, formate.

Metabolic alkalosis
Loss of H^+
— prolonged vomiting
— potassium depletion — secondary to renal tubular potassium-hydrogen exchange
— ingestion of base — old-fashioned sodium bicarbonate therapy of peptic ulcers.

Usually compensatory respiratory acidosis with hypoventilation:
— Po_2 low
— Pco_2 high.

Peak flow
— Blow into machine as hard and fast as you can.

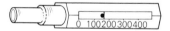

— Records in litre/min. Useful for diagnosing and observing asthma. Normal 300–500 litre/min.
— Improvement with β-agonist, e.g. isoprenaline, indicates reversible airway disease, i.e. asthma.

Spirometry
— Blow into machine (a *vitalograph*) as hard as you can — measures pattern of airflow during forced expiration.

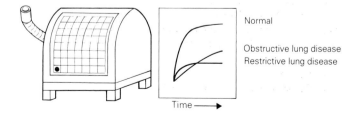

Normal

Obstructive lung disease
Restrictive lung disease

Time ⟶

— To distinguish between restrictive lung disease e.g. *emphysema*, fibrosis and obstructive lung disease, e.g. *asthma*, *chronic obstructive airways disease*.

Skin testing for allergens

Drops of a weak allergen solution are placed on to the skin, and a superficial prick of the skin, with a short lancet though the liquid, innoculates the epidermis. Special lancets coated with freeze-dried allergen can be used. A local wheal indicates an allergic response.

Carbon monoxide transfer factor

The rate of uptake of CO from inspired gas determines the lung diffusion capacity. It is reduced in alveolar diseases, e.g. *pulmonary fibrosis*.

VQ scan (V = ventilation, Q = perfusion)

Ventilation scan
— Inhalation of an isotope allows picture of airways of the lungs to be taken by a gamma camera.

Perfusion scan
— Injection of isotope into the blood stream demonstrates the blood flow in the lungs.

Mismatch of the scans is used to diagnose pulmonary embolism, i.e. air reaches all parts of the lung, while the blood does not. Matching defects occur with other lung pathology, e.g. emphysema.

N.B. A perfusion scan showing an area of ischaemia with a normal chest X-ray is generally sufficient to diagnose a pulmonary embolus. A VQ scan is needed if there is other lung pathology onX-ray, but in practice the results are difficult to interpret.

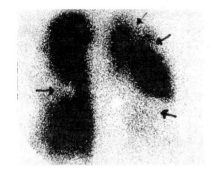

Perfusion scan; arrows mark perfusion defects.

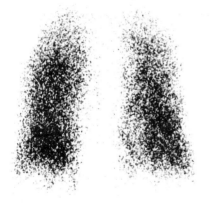

Ventilation scan; normal.

V Q scan of pulmonary embolism.

Bronchoscopy

— Rigid bronchoscopy — under general anaesthetic.
— Flexible bronchoscopy — under mild sedation, e.g. i.v. diazepam with local anaesthetic spray to pharynx and larynx. Vision by fibreoptics.

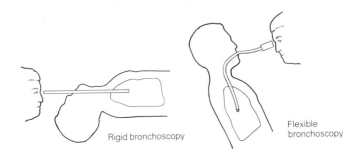

Rigid bronchoscopy

Flexible bronchoscopy

The advantages of these techniques are as follows.
— Rigid bronchoscopy. Good vision of main bronchi and carina only.
— Flexible bronchoscopy. Can be introduced to smaller bronchi.
— Biopsies can be taken by either method for neoplasms.
— Aspiration samples, sometimes after lavage with saline, can be taken for organisms and malignant cells.

Bronchogram — rarely done — a contrast medium injected into the bronchial tree to show peripheral dilated bronchi (bronchiectasis).

GASTROINTESTINAL INVESTIGATIONS

Upper GI endoscopy
A flexible fibreoptic tube is introduced into the oesophagus, stomach and duodenum after mild sedation, e.g. i.v. diazepam, with local anaesthetic to pharynx.
Direct vision of the gastrointestinal tract enables visualisation of
— oesophageal abnormalities, e.g. neoplasm, varices, oesophagitis;
— gastric-duodenal abnormalities, e.g. neoplasm, ulcers, gastritis, gastic atrophy.

Endoscopic retrograde cholangio-pancreatography (ERCP): through an endoscope, under direct vision, a tube is inserted through the ampulla and introduction of a radio-opaque contrast medium allows X-ray visualisation of:

— biliary tree, for stones, tumours, strictures, irregularities;
— pancreatic ducts, for chronic pancreatitis, dilated ducts or distortion from a tumour.

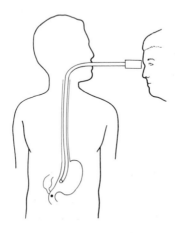

The endoscope can be used for surgery, including sphincterotomy of ampulla for removal of gallstones in the bile duct, introduction of a rigid tube, a stent, through a constricting tumour to allow biliary drainage.

Proctoscopy, sigmoidoscopy, colonoscopy (see p. 132)

Barium swallow, meal, enema

Barium is drunk (swallow for oesophagus, meal for stomach/duodenum) or introduced rectally (enema) or via a catheter into the duodenum (small-bowel enema).

X-rays are taken with barium coating the mucosa. Air may be introduced to distend organs and to give 'double contrast' films. Outlines physical abnormalities
— strictures, e.g. fibrosis, carcinomas
— filling defects, e.g. polyps, carcinomas
— craters, e.g. ulcers, diverticulae
— mucosal irregularities
    — mucosal folds radiating from peptic ulcer

— clefts in Crohn's disease of colon
— featureless mucosa of early ulcerative colitis
— islands of mucosa in severe ulcerative colitis.

An irregularity on a single film needs to be seen on other views before an abnormality is confirmed, as peristalsis or gut contents can mimic defects.

Cholecystogram

An initial plain film to show radio-opaque gallstones. A radio-opaque contrast is taken by mouth, excreted by the liver and concentrated in the gall bladder.

— Cholesterol gallstones give filling defects in the gall bladder.
— Non-visualisation of the gall bladder may occur in some normal subjects, from a stone in the cystic duct or subsequent fibrosis.

Cholangiogram

Intravenous contrast is excreted promptly to show bile ducts.

— widened if obstruction
— may show gallstones in bile duct.

Hydrogen breath test

Oral lactulose is given, and excess gut flora in the small bowel or blind loop causes prompt metabolism to provide exhaled hydrogen.

RENAL INVESTIGATIONS

Urine testing

Testing the urine is part of the routine physical examination. It is most simply done using one of the combination dip sticks.

• Dip the stick in the urine and compare the colours with the key at the times specified. Of particular interest are:

— pH
— protein content (**N.B.** Does not detect Bence Jones Protein)
— ketones
— glucose
— bilirubin
— urobilinogen
— blood/haemoglobin.

Urine microscopy

Urine may be viewed centrifuged or uncentrifuged. Centrifuging concentrates the formed elements but may disrupt fragile ones.

• Spin a small volume at 1000–1500 r.p.m. for 3 minutes, pour off all but the last 0.5 ml and resuspend the deposit in this by shaking the tube.

• Put a drop on a slide and view through a cover slip.

• A rough quantitative guide is made by counting the formed elements per high power field.

	Normal number/high power field (Centrifuged)
Red cells (small round)	< 1
White cells (lobulated nuclei)	5
Epithelial cells (Single nuclei, round)	Suggest contamination
Casts	0
— Hyaline ⎤ recognised — Red cell ⎬ with — Granular ⎦ practice	
Bacteria	0

Urine may be Gram stained. It is best to Gram stain the centrifuged sediment. The Gram stain can also be used for pus.

• Apply specimen to slide and fix by heating.
• Stain with Methyl Violet for 1 minute.
• Wash with iodine and stand for 1 minute.
• Wash with water.
• Decolorise with acetone *briefly*.
• Counterstain: neutral red for 2 minutes.
• Wash with water and dry.

Creatinine clearance

Precise measurements of the *Glomerular Filtration Rate* are made isotopically, e.g. Cr EDTA clearance. The creatinine clearance is easier to organise although less accurate.

• Collect a blood sample for plasma creatinine.

• Collect 24-hour urine sample for creatinine.

Formula $\dfrac{U \times V}{P \times T}$

$$\dfrac{\text{Urine (Creatinine)}}{\underset{(\mu\text{mol})}{\text{Plasma (Creatinine)}}} \times \dfrac{\underset{(\text{ml}) \times 10^3}{\text{Urine vol.}}}{\underset{(\text{mins})}{\text{Duration collection}}} = \text{Clearance (ml/min)}$$

Normal value 80–120 ml/min.

Intravenous pyelogram
An initial plain film to show renal or ureteric stones. Contrast medium is injected i.v. concentrated in the kidney and excreted.
• 'Nephrogram' phase — kidneys are outlined
    — observe position, size, shape, filling defects, e.g. tumour.
• Excretion phase — renal pelvis
    — Renal papillae may be lost from chronic pyelonephritis.
    — Calyces blunted from hydronephrosis.
    — Pelvi-ureteric obstruction — large pelvis, normal ureters.
• Ureters — observe position — Displaced by other pathology?
    — Size — dilated from obstruction or recent infection
    — Irregularities — may be contractions and need to be checked in sequential films.

NEUROLOGICAL INVESTIGATIONS

Electroencephalogram
Multiple electrodes are applied to the scalp and brain waves are recorded using a sophisticated amplifier.

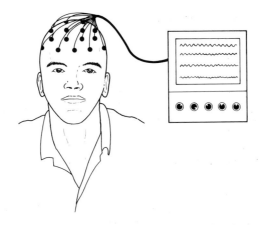

The main value of this technique is in showing episodes of abnormal waves compatible with epilepsy. Large normal variation makes interpretation difficult.

Lumbar puncture

A needle is introduced between the lumbar vertebrae, through the dura into the subarachnoid space, and cerebrospinal fluid is obtained for examination.

Normal cerebrospinal fluid is completely clear.

The major diagnostic value of this technique is in:
— subarachnoid haemmorhage — uniformly red, whereas blood from a 'traumatic' tap is in the first specimen;
— xanthochromia — yellow stain from haemoglobin breakdown;
— meningitis — pyogenic, turbid fluid, white cells, organisms on culture, low glucose and raised protein;
— raised pressure may indicate a tumour.

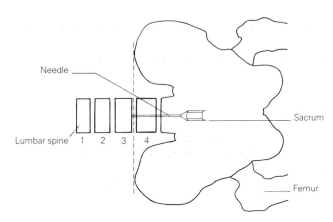

Lumbar puncture needle: between L3, L4 in line with the superior posterior iliac crest

HAEMATOLOGICAL INVESTIGATIONS

Blood film
- Apply a drop of blood to one end of a slide placed on a level surface.
- Hold the narrow edge of a second slide against the drop and allow the blood to spread across (a).

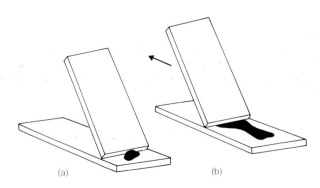

(a)   (b)

- With the second slide inclined at 45° draw it along the first, spreading the blood (b).
- Dry the film in air and stain using Leischman's stain.
- View under oil immersion.

Leischman's stain
- Make a blood film.
- Cover film with Leischman's stain.
- After 1 minute add twice the quantity of distilled water.
- After 7 minutes pour off the mixture.
- Cover with distilled water for a further 2 minutes
- Pour off and blot dry.

Differential count
- Count 100 white cells and work out the percentage of each type.

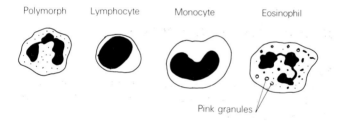

Polymorph   Lymphocyte   Monocyte   Eosinophil

Pink granules

Bone marrow
After insertion of local anaesthetic by the periosteum, a needle is inserted into the bone marrow, usually the sternum. The aspirate is examined for red and white cell precursors, and is useful in the diagnosis of:
- — leukaemias
- — myeloma
- — megaloblastic marrow — vitamin B_{12} deficiency.

HYPER AND HYPOGLYCAEMIA

Blood glucose

Colorimetric methods

Several proprietary glucose-oxidase colour strips are available. Examples include Ames and Boehringer strips for use with meters, or visual use. Make sure the strips have been kept in a sealed container.

• Prick finger with a lancet, and squeeze finger tip to produce drop of blood.

• Put one large drop of blood on to the pad on the strip — a smear will *not* do.

• Time precisely for 1 minute (second hand of watch or digital watch).
  — Ames Strips: wash off blood, preferably with a wash bottle, and read strip immediately.
  — Boehringer Strips: wipe off blood using cotton wool or tissue paper, wait one more minute before reading strip.

• Use a colorimeter for a precise reading, particularly in the hypoglycaemic range.

Amperometric methods

Some machines give a direct current output from a glucose-oxidase strip
  — Exactech: after applying blood to the strip, the result is shown within half a minute.

Chapter 11
The 12-Lead Electrocardiogram

THE ECG

The ECG tracings arise from the electrical changes, depolarisation and repolarisation, that accompany muscle contraction. With knowledge of the relative position of the leads to the electrodes, the ECG tracings provide direct information of the cardiac muscle and its activity.

Six *'standard'* leads, I, II, III, aVR, aVL, aVF, are recorded from the limb electrodes (aV = augmented voltage), and examine the heart from different directions.

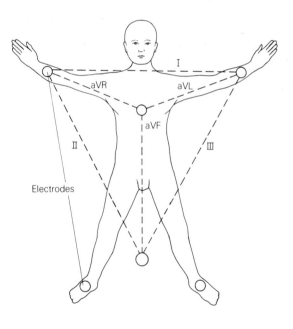

The standard leads examine the heart in the *vertical* plane

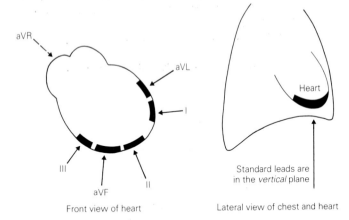

Front view of heart

Lateral view of chest and heart

Six chest leads, 'V leads', attached by suction electrodes to the chest wall, are all in the **horizontal** plane.

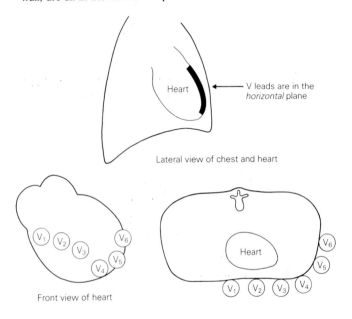

Lateral view of chest and heart

Front view of heart

Obstruction of arteries gives appropriate specific patterns of ischaemia.

Left anterior descending coronary artery — *anterior ischaemia or infarct* (V_1–V_6).

Circumflex coronary artery — *lateral ischaemia or infarct* (I, aVL).

Right coronary artery — *inferior ischaemia or infarct* (II, III, aVF).

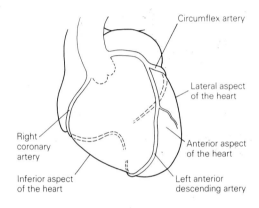

Every ECG tracing must first be standardised by making sure the 1 mV mark deviates the pointer ten small squares on the paper.

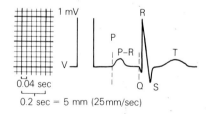

P   = atrial depolarisation
QRS = ventricular depolarisation
T   = repolarisation

All cardiac muscle has tendency to depolarisation leading to excitation and contraction.

Initial electrical discharge from SA node (under influence of sympathetic and parasympathetic control) spreads to atrio-ventricular (AV) node and via bundle of His to ventricles.

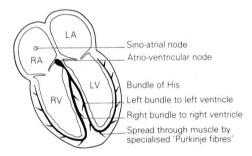

LA

RA

LV

RV

Sino-atrial node
Atrio-ventricular node

Bundle of His
Left bundle to left ventricle
Right bundle to right ventricle
Spread through muscle by specialised 'Purkinje fibres'

The deflection of the ECG tracing indicates the average direction of all muscle activity at each moment.

Depolarisation spreads:

— towards lead — ECG tracing moves up the paper.
— away from lead — tracing moves down paper.

P wave
- Depolarisation spreads from SA node through the atrial muscle fibres to AV node
- best seen in lead II
- usually small, as atria are small.

Normal P wave < 2.5 mm high, < 2.5 mm wide

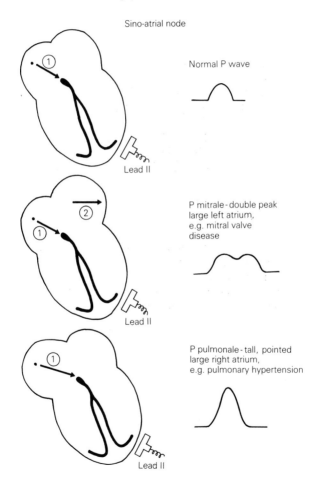

Sino-atrial node

Normal P wave

Lead II

P mitrale - double peak large left atrium, e.g. mitral valve disease

Lead II

P pulmonale - tall, pointed large right atrium, e.g. pulmonary hypertension

Lead II

ORS complex

The QRS deflections have a standard nomenclature:

Q — any initial deflection downwards

R — any deflection upwards whether or not a preceding Q

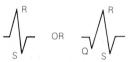

S — any deflection downwards after an R wave whether or not a preceding Q

The QRS in the V leads

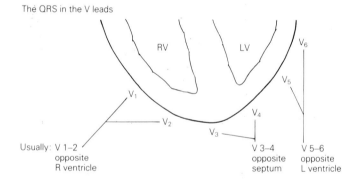

The septum depolarises first from left to right.

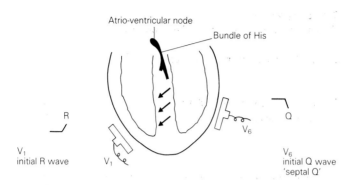

The ventricles then depolarise from inside outwards. The large left ventricle then normally dominates.

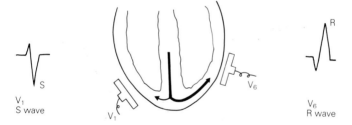

The 'transition point' where R and S are equal is the position of the septum.

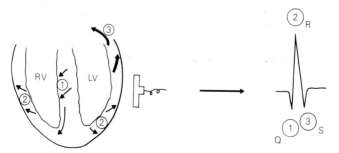

V_6 S wave after R wave as depolarisation spreads around ventricle away from V_6.

Left ventricle hypertrophy

V_5 or V_6 — R wave >25 mm
V_1 or V_2 — S wave deep
Tallest R wave + deepest S wave
>35 mm.

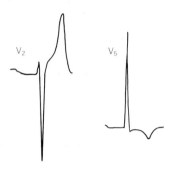

S_{V_2} = 23 mm + R_{V_5} = 25 mm = 48 mm

— Voltage changes on their own are not enough — thin people with thin rib cage can have big complexes
— obese people small complexes
— Also look for R wave in V_1 — rotation to right of transition point axis deviation
— T wave inversion in V_5, V_6, termed left ventricular 'strain pattern', indicates marked hypertrophy.

Right ventricle hypertrophy

The left ventricle is no longer dominant
V_1 — R wave > S wave
V_6 — deep S wave.

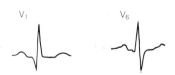

— Also look for — right axis deviation
          — peaked P of right atrial hypertrophy
          — T wave inversion in V_2 and V_3 — right ventricular 'strain pattern'.

Myocardial infarct — dead muscle

Pathological Q wave
- Full thickness infarct of ventricle.

  Width = or > 0.04 seconds (one small square).

  Depth > 1/3 height of R wave.

  Smaller Q waves are physiological from septum depolarisation.
- As ventricles depolarise from inside, an electrode in the ventricle cavity would record contraction as Q wave.
- Through 'dead' window, this is seen as if from 'inside' the heart, i.e. the depolarisation of the far ventricle wall away from the electrode gives a negative deflection.

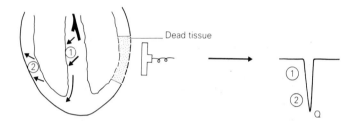

Myocardial ischaemia

Damaged but potentially salvagable myocardium

Raised ST segment
- ST segment — normally within 0.5 mm of isoelectric line
- ST elevation in V_1 and V_2 may be normal — high 'takeoff' of j point.

Normal baseline:

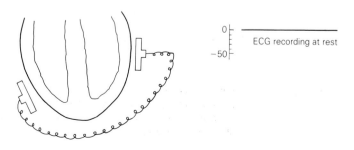

Resting myocardial cell — potential approximately − 90 mV. In an injured cell, failing cell membrane only allows potential of perhaps − 40 mV.

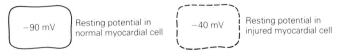

If two electrodes record from different areas of the resting heart, one normal and one injured, a galvanometer would register − 50 mV (i.e. the difference between − 90 mV and − 40 mV). This depresses the baseline below normal over the injured area, although this cannot be recognised until after QRS complex.

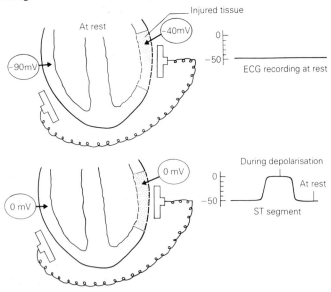

Raised ST segment:
— acute ischaemic injury of ventricle
— pericarditis
— normal athletes
— normal West Indians.

Time Sequence of onset of ECG changes in infarction

Approximate time of onset after chest pain		ECG changes
Immediately	1. May be normal	ECG may be normal. Occasionally ST segment changes occur immediately pain develops, or even before
0–2 hours	2.	ST segments rise — occluded artery → injury pattern
3–8 hours	3.	Injured tissue remains Some dies (Q waves = Death) Some improves to become ischaemic only 　(T wave inversion) Full infarct pattern: — Q waves — raised ST segments — inverted T waves
8–24 hours	4.	Injured tissue either dies → Q wave or improves to ischaemia → ST segments disappear Inverted T waves remain
After 1–2 days	5.	Ischaemia disappears T waves upright again Q waves usually remain, as dead tissue will not come alive again

Q waves may disappear if scarred tissue contracts.

Ischaemic myocardium

Reduced oxygen supply to muscle:
— ST depression
— T wave inversion
— Occasionally tall pointed T wave.

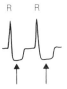 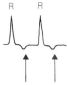 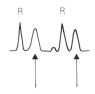

Depressed ST segment   T wave inversion   Tall sharp pointed T waves

QRS axis

— The direction of depolarisation of the heart is sometimes helpful in diagnosis.
— Note the axis deviation on its own is rarely significant but alerts you to look for right or left ventricular hypertrophy.
— Look at the standard leads for the most equiphasic QRS complex (R and S equal). The axis is approximately at right angles to this in the direction of the most positive standard lead (largest R wave).

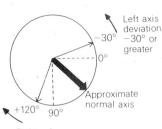 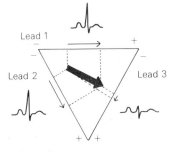

Pattern recognition.

Left axis deviation

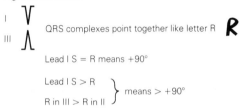

I

III

QRS complexes part like arms of letter L

Lead II S = R means $-30°$

Lead II S > R
S in III > R in I } means $> -30°$

Right axis deviation

I

III

QRS complexes point together like letter R

Lead I S = R means $+90°$

Lead I S > R
R in III > R in II } means $> +90°$

QRS complex
Normal if width < 0.12 second (3 small squares).
If > 0.12 second — bundle branch block.
Right bundle branch block (RBBB) — M pattern in V_1
Left bundle branch block (LBBB)   — M pattern in V_6
— throughout ECG, slurred ST segment and T wave inversion opposite to major deflection of QRS.
An inverted T wave in bundle branch block (QRS > 0.12 second) is not significant on its own.

An apparently wide QRS complex, < 0.12 second wide — partial bundle branch block or inter-ventricular conduction defect.

Left bundle branch block
— Lead V_6 — depolarisation of septal muscle from right bundle gives positive deflection;
— right heart depolarisation gives negative deflection;
— left heart depolarisation gives positive deflection.

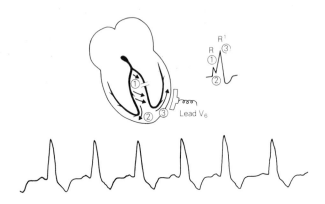

— Standard leads — left axis deviation as impulse spreads from right
bundle up to left ventricle;
— also occurs if only anterior fascicle of left
bundle blocked;
— left anterior hemiblock.

Right bundle branch block
— Lead V_1 — depolarisation of septal muscle from left bundle gives
positive deflection;
— left heart depolarisation gives negative deflection;
— right heart depolarisation gives positive deflection.

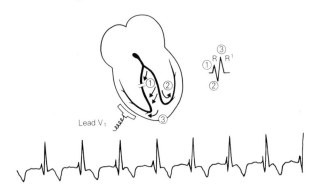

— Standard leads — axis usually normal, as depends on large muscle
mass of left ventricle;
— if right bundle branch block is associated with
left axis block of anterior fascicle of left
bundle — bifascicular block.
— All heart is being excited via remaining posterior fascicle of left bundle.

Arrhythmias
— Ectopics
— Tachycardias
— Bradycardias.

Ectopics
Atrial ectopics
Ectopic focus anywhere in atria.
Depolarisation spreads across atrium to AV node like any normal beat.

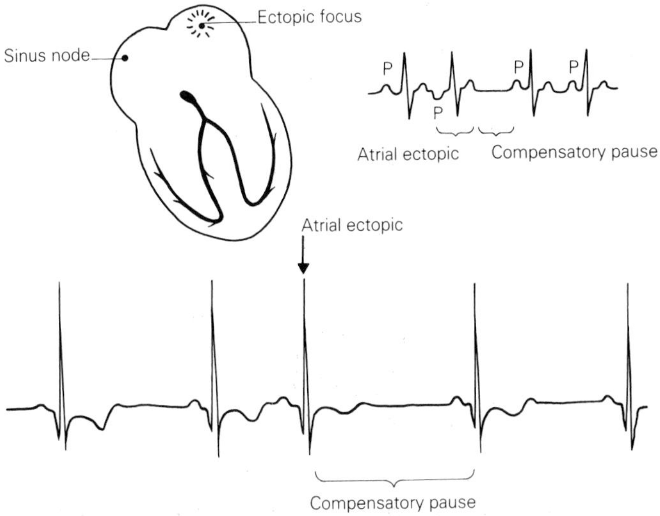

Sinus node

Ectopic focus

P   P   P

P

Atrial ectopic   Compensatory pause

Atrial ectopic

Compensatory pause

— P wave abnormal shape

— normal QRS complex.

The atrial ectopic focus must fire early — or would be entrained by normal excitation.

— appears early on rhythm strip

— followed by compensatory pause — waiting for normal SA node cycle.

Junctional ectopics

Ectopic at AV node; no P wave.

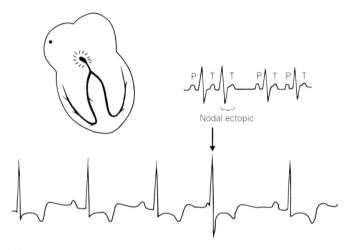

Junctional or nodal; ectopic at AV node; no P wave

Ventricular ectopics

Ectopic anywhere in ventricles.

Depolarisation occurs first in that ventricle then spreads to other ventricle

— no P wave

— wide complex

— bundle branch block pattern — left focus — RBBB pattern

— right focus — LBBB pattern.

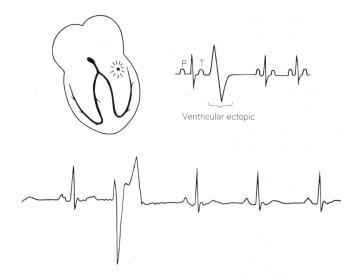

Ventricular ectopic

Many patients have innocent ventricular ectopics that disappear on exercise, and there is no need to treat them when found accidently. If R on T occurs (R wave of ventricular ectopic occurs on the downstroke of the T wave of an ordinary beat) ventricular tachycardia may be triggered.

Tachycardias
Re-entry
Re-entry is the most common mechanism. Assumes two conduction pathways lead to ventricles. Normally conduction passes equally quickly down both pathways.

Problems arise when one pathway recovers more slowly than the other. When this happens the next conduction passes down only one pathway.

Conduction subsequently passes retrogradely up the other pathway which is no longer refractory. This pathway then becomes refractory while the first pathway conducts again and the impulse races round the pathways to give a tachycardia.

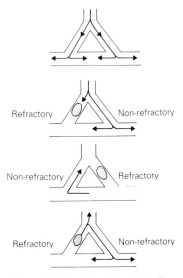

The mechanism of re-entry tachycardias

Wolff–Parkinson–White syndrome (W–P–W syndrome)

This is the classical re-entry arrhythmia. There are two separate pathways from the atria to the ventricles.

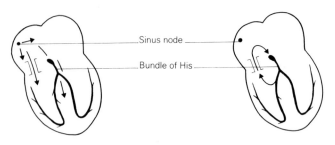

Normal depolarisation
in the W–P–W syndrome

Tachycardia produced via
accessory pathway in
W–P–W syndrome

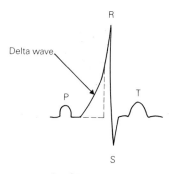

The QRS complex in
W-P-W syndrome

Atrial fibrillation

The electrical impulse and contraction travels around the atria
— 'bag of worms' quivering atria
— Irregular little waves on ECG — best seen V_1.
When it first develops, often 150 + and fibrillation waves difficult to see.

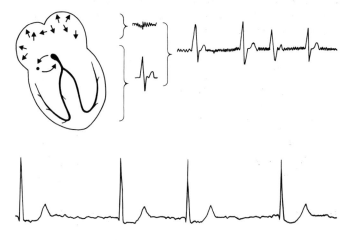

The ECG of atrial fibrillation

— AV node fires irregularly
— normal QRS complexes.
    If irregular rate, no P waves, normal QRS — likely to be atrial
    fibrillation
Digoxin is still the drug of choice — it decreases transmission of
impulses down Bundle of His.

Atrial flutter

Atria contract very rapidly, 200–250/minutes^2, giving 'saw-tooth
pattern', but the ventricles only respond to every second or third or
fourth contraction (2:1, 3:1, 4:1 block).

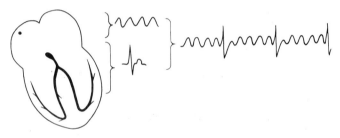

Treated with digoxin, normally changes to atrial fibrillation.

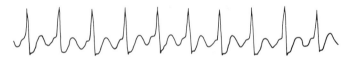

The ECG of atrial flutter 2:1

Supraventricular tachycardia (SVT)

— Arises near AV node, 170/minute or more, regular.
— Complexes are identical, normal width or wide if also bundle
    branch block.
— common in young patients (20–30 years).
— Rarely represents heart disease.
— Sudden onset and finish.
— Last few minutes to several hours.
— May be tired, lightheaded uncomfortable.
— In older patients SVTs more likely to represent heart disease.

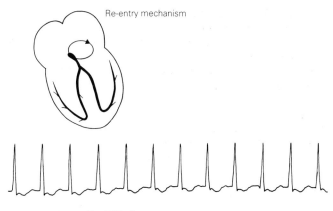

Re-entry mechanism

The ECG of supraventricular tachycardia.

Vagal stimulation (rubbing carotid sinus) can terminate attack.

Ventricular tachycardia
— Potentially dangerous rhythm which can develop into VF.
— Rapid but not as fast as SVT (usually less than 170/minute).

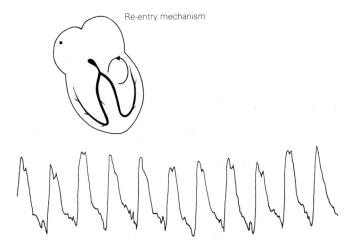

Re-entry mechanism

The ECG of ventricular tachycardia.

— Often slightly irregular.
— Patient often looks collapsed.
— Always wide PR interval — left bundle block pattern — right focus
— Right bundle block pattern — left focus

Treatment is with lignocaine 100 mg i.v. stat with transfer of the patient to hospital.

Bradycardias
— Pulse rate < 60/minute.

Sinus
— Normal P wave and QRS complexes.

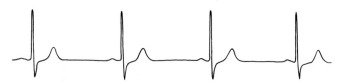

The ECG of sinus bradycardia

Causes:
— Athlete
— Beta-blockers
— Hypothyroidism
— Raised intracranial pressure
— Pain with vagal response — dental pain
      — glaucoma
      — biliary colic.

Heart block
1st degree
— PR interval (beginning of P wave to beginning of QRS complex) > 0.22 second (5½ little squares).
— Depolarisation delayed in the region of AV node.

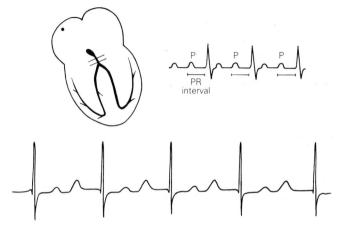

The ECG of first-degree heart block

Wenkebach

In a cycle of three or four beats the PR interval gradually lengthens until a P wave appears on its own with no QRS complex. The cycle then repeats itself.

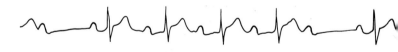

Gradually increasing PR interval until a QRS is dropped

Wenkebach block

2.1 Block

The QRS complexes only respond to every other P wave, i.e. every other P wave has no QRS complex.

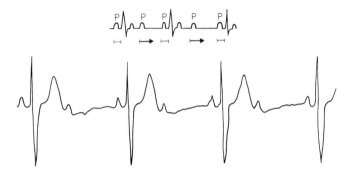

Second-degree heart block

Complete heart block
  — No relation between P waves and QRS complex.
  — Inherent ventricular rate about 40/minute.
  — QRS complex abnormal as it arises in a ventricular focus.

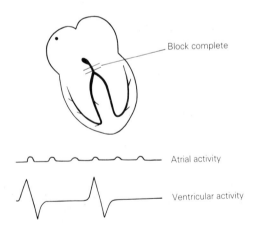

Block complete

Atrial activity

Ventricular activity

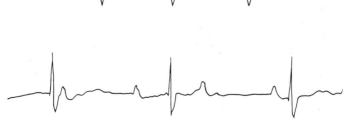

The ECG of complete heart block.

LOOKING AT THE ECG

Examine logically, reading complexes from left to right.

- Rhythm
  - Sinus rhythm ± ectopics. Ignore sinus arrhythmia.
  - Regular — slow complete heart block
    - sinus bradycardia
    - fast sinus tachycardia
    - supraventricular tachycardia
    - ventricular tachycardia
    - regular atrial flutter.
  - Irregular — atrial fibrillation
    - atrial tachycardia with varying block.
- *Rate*

Add up the number of large squares between two successive beats. Divide into 300. For example:

$$\frac{300}{5 \text{ large squares}} = 60/\text{minute}$$

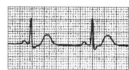

1½ squares	= 200/minute	3½	= 85/minute
2	= 150/minute	4	= 75/minute
2½	= 120/minute	5	= 60/minute
3	= 100/minite	6	= 50/minute

Simple formula does not work for irregular rhythm — then add up number of complexes in 6 seconds (sometimes marked on the paper) and multiply by 10.

- *Complex shape* — brief guide
  - P wave: abnormal shape — atrial ectopics, p mitrale, p. pulmonale. — 0.10–0.22 second (2½ –5½ squares).
  - PR interval: prolonged — > 0.22 second: First degree heart block — < 0.1 second: Wolff–Parkinson–White syndrome.
  - QRS complex: large Q wave — full thickness infarct?
    wide QRS   > 0.12 second: branch block
    R wave   if large: ventrical hypertrophy?
  - ST segment: elevated or depressed — ischaemia or other causes?
  - T wave: if inverted — ischaemia or other causes?

In summary, particularly look for:
- Abnormal rhythm.
- Abnormal rate.
- Abnormal QRS — especially ischaemia, infarct, hypertrophy.

Chapter 12
Interpretation of Investigations

SENSITIVITY, SPECIFICITY AND EFFICIENCY

These terms have specific meanings which indicate the clinical usefulness of investigations. Sensitivity and specificity assess the frequency of results in relation to the correct answers.

		Correct diagnosis	
		+	−
Test	+	true positive	false positive
result	−	false negative	true negative

Sensitivity — how often the correct postive answer is obtained in those who have the disease

$$= \frac{\text{True positive}}{\text{True positive} + \text{false negative}} \quad \text{i.e.}$$

It also expresses the likelihood that a negative test result correctly indicates disease is not present: 95% sensitivity means five false negatives in 100 patients with the disease.

Specificity — how often the correct negative answer is obtained in those who do not have the disease

$$= \frac{\text{True negative}}{\text{True negative} + \text{false positive}} \quad \text{i.e.}$$

It also expresses the likelihood that a positive rest result will correctly indicate disease: 90% specificity means 10 false positives in 100 subjects tested who do not have the disease.

> Thus a large heart on X-ray is a fairly sensitive test for severe mitral regurgitation (most patients with mitral regurgitation have a large heart) but it is not a specific test (because many heart diseases produce a large heart).

Efficiency — how often the investigation gives the correct answer

$$= \frac{\text{True positive} + \text{true negative}}{\text{All tests}} \quad \text{i.e.}$$

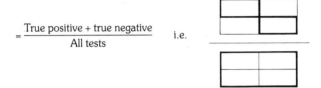

INTERPRETATION

The reliance put on the result of an investigation depends on the *a priori* chance of the result being abnormal. Thus a high plasma calcium in a woman with breast cancer would be taken to indicate either bone metastases or the non-metatastic hypercalcaemia (due to tumour production of a parathormone like peptide), whereas a similar value in an apparently normal medical student would be regarded as being a false positive until it were re-checked. Where the prior probability of an event is known, Bayes theorem can be used to calculate the current probability. The prevalence of an abnormality in the population therefore assists interpretation of an individual patient's results. Please note the difference between prevalence and incidence.

PREVALENCE AND INCIDENCE

Prevalence — the number of cases of a disease in a designated population, e.g. 10% of males aged 40–60 years.

Incidence — the number of new cases during a specific period, e.g. 10 per 100 000 population per annum.

Chapter 13
Laboratory Results — Normal Values

Normal ranges are the most frequently used reference interval. For some situations, *specific diagnostic reference intervals* are appropriate, e.g. twice normal value of plasma creatine kinase for diagnosing Duchenne muscular dystrophy. *Action limits* can be set which aid decision taking, e.g. a cholesterol value in the upper normal range (> 5.5 mmol/litre) may require therapy. *Patient-specific reference intervals* are sometimes required for therapeutic purposes, e.g. specific glucose control criteria for different diabetic patients.

NORMAL VALUES

Methods and their normal ranges vary from laboratory-to-laboratory and according to the sex and age distribution of the reference healthy population. The following results are a general guide and may not be apposite for your laboratory.

HAEMATOLOGY

	Male	Female
Haemoglobin	13.5–18.0 g/dl	11.5–16.0 g/dl
Packed cell volume (PCV)	40–54%	37–47%
Red cell count	$4.5–6.5 \times 10^{12}$/litre	$3.9–5.6 \times 10^{12}$/litre
Mean cell volume (MCV)		81–100 fl
Mean cell haemoglobin		27–32 pg
Mean cell haemoglobin concentration		32–36 g/dl
Reticulocyte count		0.8–2%
White cell count		$4.0–11.0 \times 10^{9}$/litre

Platelets	$150–400 \times 10^9$/litre
Prothrombin time	10–14 seconds
Erythrocyte sedimentation rate (ESR).	

Westergren at 1 hour

| Male | Female |
| 0–10 mm | 0–15 mm |

(Higher values of ESR may occur in normal elderly patients)

CEREBROSPINAL FLUID

Glucose	2.8–4.2 mmol/litre
Pressure	70–180 mmH$_2$O
Protein	0.15–0.45 g/litre
Cells	0–5 white cells
	0 red cells

CLINICAL CHEMISTRY (IN SI UNITS)

Blood

Acid phosphatase (total)	1–5 iu/litre
Acid phosphatase (prostatic)	0–1 iu/litre
Albumin	35–50 g/litre
Alkaline phosphatase (adult)	30–300 iu/litre
Amylase	25–180 Somogyi units/dl
Anion gap	7–16 mmol/litre
Bicarbonate	24–30 mmol/litre
Bilirubin (total)	3–17 μmol/litre
Bilirubin in babies (toxic value)	>200 μmol/litre
Bilirubin (conjugated)	0–5 μmol/litre
Calcium	2.12–2.65 mmol/litre
Carcinoembryonic antigen	0–9 μmol/litre
Chloride	95–105 mmol/litre
Cholesterol	3.9–7.8 mmol/litre

Copper	12–26 µmol/litre
Cortisol (0900 hr)	450–700 nmol/litre
Cortisol (midnight)	80–280 nmol/litre
C-peptide (fasting — interpret with glucose value)	0.2–0.8 nmol/litre
Creatine phosphokinase (men)	24–175 iu/litre
Creatine phosphokinase (women)	24–195 iu/litre
Creatinine	70–150 µmol/litre
Ferritin (women)	12–150 µmol/litre
Ferritin (men)	15–200 µmol/litre
Alpha fetoprotein	0–14 kU/litre
Folate (serum)	2.1–18 µg/litre
Folate (red cell)	160–640 µg/litre
Follicle stimulating hormone	2–8 U/litre
Gamma glutamyl transpeptidase (women)	7–35 iu/litre
Gamma glutamyl transpeptidase (men)	11–51 iu/litre
Glucose (plasma, fasting)	3.8–5.5 mmol/litre
IgG	7.2–19 g/litre
IgA	0.8–5.9 g/litre
IgM	0.5–2.0 g/litre
IgE	<120 kU/litre
Insulin (fasting — interpret with glucose value)	2–13 mU/litre
Iron (women)	11–30 µmol/litre
Iron (men)	14–31 µmol/litre
Iron binding capacity	54–75 µmol/litre
Lactate (fasting)	0.6–2.0 mmol/litre
Lactate dehydrogenase	70–170 iu/litre
Lead (blood)	<0.12 µmol/litre
Luteinising hormone	3–8 U/litre
Magnesium	0.75–1.05 mmol/litre
Osmolality	278–305 mOsm/kg
Phosphate	0.8–1.45 mmol/litre
Potassium	3.5–5.0 mmol/litre
Prolactin (women)	<600 mU/litre

Prolactin (men)	<400 mU/litre
Sodium	134–145 mmol/litre
Testosterone (women)	1.0–2.5 nmol/litre
Testosterone (men)	9–42 nmol/litre
Total protein	60–80 g/litre
Transaminase (GOT, AST)	5–35 iu/litre
Transaminase (GPT, ALT)	5–45 iu/litre
Triglyceride (fasting)	0.6–1.9 mmol/litre
Thyroxine	70–140 nmol/litre
Thyroxine (free)	9–25 pmol/litre
Triiodothyronine	1.0–3.0 nmol/litre
Urate (men)	<480 µmol/litre
Urate (women)	<390 µmol/litre
Urea	2.5–6.7 mmol/litre
Vitamin B12	150–750 ng/litre

24-hour urine

Calcium	2.5–7.5 mmol/day
5HIAA,5–OH indole acetic acid	10–42 µmol/day
Cortisol	28–280 nmol/day
HMMA, OH methylmandelic acid	10–35 µmol/day
HVA, Homo vanillic acid	<82 µmol/day
Metanephrine	<5.5 µmol/day
Potassium	40–120 mmol/day
Protein	<80 mg/day
Sodium	100–250 mmol/day
Urea	250–500 mmol/day

Drugs in serum

The following are usual therapeutic ranges. The value related to the time of ingestion is crucial for some drugs, e.g. plasma paracetamol >1.0 mmol/litre gives a risk of liver damage but the decision interval of the plasma level for therapy decreases with time after an overdose.

Amiodarone — before dose	0.6–2.5 mg/litre
Carbamazepine — before dose	34–51 µmol/litre

Carbon monoxide — non-smoker	0–2%
Carbon monoxide — smoker	0–5%
Digoxin — at least 6 hours after last dose	1.0–2.0 µg/litre
Disopyramide — before dose	2.0–5.0 mg/dl
Epanutin — before dose	40–80 µmol/litre
Ethosuximide — before dose	250–710 µmol/litre
Lithium	0.5–1.5 mmol/litre
Salicylate	0.4–2.5 mmol/litre
Theophylline — before dose	55–110 µmol/litre
Valproate — before dose	0.3–0.7 mmol/litre

Toxic levels

Barbiturate — potentially fatal	
— short acting	5 µmol/litre
— medium acting	105 µmol/litre
— long acting	215 µmol/litre
Ethanol (physiological <0.2 nmol/litre)	
— legal limit for driving	<17.4 nmol/litre
Paracetamol	
— at anytime	>1.0 mmol/litre
— at 12 hours	>0.5 mmol/litre

Miscellaneous

Sweat chloride	6–40 mmol/litre
Foecal fat	<18 mmol/day

Index

'a' wave of JVP   38
Abdomen, examination   65, 109
Abdominal pain   9
Abdominal X-ray   135
Abducens nerve   86
Acalculia   79
Accessory nerve   91
Accommodation reflex   85
Acromegaly   28
Activities of daily living (ADL)   121
Addison's disease   28
Aegophony   60
Agnosia   79
Alcohol   23
Allergens, skin testing for   148
Allergies   14
Alveolitis
    allergic   64
    fibrosing   21, 60
Ames strips   158
Amperometric methods, blood
        glucose   158
Anaemia   23, 34, 35
Angina pectoris   7
Angiography
    background subtraction   137
    coronary   144
Angular stomatitis   65
Ankle   98
    reflexes   99
    swelling   8
Ankylosing spondylitis   32
Anxiety   11
Aorta, abdominal   70
Aortic area   40
Aortic incompetence   34, 36, 43, 44,
        45, 50
Aortic stenosis   34, 36, 39, 43, 44,
        45, 49
Apex beat   57
    hearing   39
    sustained   39
    tapping   40
Aphasia   78
Appendicitis   75
Appetite   7
Apraxia   79
Arcus senilis   23

Argyll–Robertson pupils   85
Arms   93
    basic examination   110
Arrhythmias   173
Arterial blood gases and pH   145
Arteriography   136
Arthralgia   12, 30
Arthritis   12, 30
Arthropathy   30
Asbestos   62
Asthma   63
Atheroma   36
Atherosclerosis   34, 35
Athetosis   92
Atrial ectopics   173
Atrial fibrillation   27, 34, 38, 177
Atrial flutter   178
Atrial septal defect   50
Attention   80
Auditory nerve   90
Auscultation   19, 40, 59
Austin Flint murmur   50

Babinski reflex   100
Background subtraction
        angiography   137
Balanitis   73
Barium swallow, meal, enema   151
Barrel chest   56
Barthel index of ADL   121
Basal crepitations   47
Basic examinations   108
Bisferiens pulse   34
Bitemporal hemianopia   28, 83
Bjerrum screen   83
Bladder, distended   97
Blindness, unilateral   83
Blood   188
    differential count   157
    film   156
    glucose   158
Blood pressure   35
    diastolic   35
    systolic   35
Blue bloater   63
Boehringer strips   158
Bone marrow   157

Bowel
  habit   9
  sounds   71
Bradycardia   180
Breasts   26
Breathlessness   8
Breath sounds
  bronchial   59
  vesicular   59
Bronchiectasis   9, 21, 55, 64
Bronchogram   151
Bronchoscopy   132, 149
Bruit
  arterial   71
  hepatic   72
Bundle branch block
  left   171
  right   171, 172

Cancer   25
Cannon waves   38
Canter rhythm   42
Carbon dioxide retention   35
Carbon monoxide transfer factor   148
Carcinoma, bronchus   9, 21, 55
Cardiac catheterization   143
Cardiac isotopic scans   144
Cardiological investigations   139
Cardiovascular system   108
  examination   33
  history   7–9
CAT scan   135
Cerebellar dysfunction   93, 107
Cerebellar gait   104
Cerebrospinal fluid   188
Charcot's joint   30
Chemosis   27
Chest
  examination   55
  pain   7
  X-ray   133
Cheyne Stokes respiration   55
Cholangiogram   152
Cholecystitis   75
Cholecystogram   152
Chorea   92
Chronic myeloid leukaemia   69
Cirrhosis of liver   21, 69, 74
'Clasp knife' movement   94
Clinical chemistry, normal values   188
Clinical investigations   130
Clonus   97, 99
Clubbing   21, 33, 55, 65
'Coffee grounds' vomit   9
Cognitive function   120

'Cogwheel' rigidity   94
Collapse of lung   58, 61
Colonoscopy   132
Colorimetric methods, blood
      glucose   158
Colposcopy   133
Computerised axial tomography   135
Confusion   65, 78, 123
Congenital heart disease, cyanotic   21
Congestive cardiac failure   69
Conjunctiva   23
Conscious level   77
Consolidation   58, 61
Constrictive pericarditis   34, 37
Coordination   93, 98
Cornea   23
Corneal reflex   88
Coronary angiography   144
Cortical sensation   105
Cough   8
Crackles   60
Cranial nerves   81
  basic examination   110
Creatinine clearance   153
Cremasteric reflex   97
Crepitations   60
Crepitus   31
Crohn's disease   21
Cushing's syndrome   29, 66
Cyanosis   22, 33
Cyst   25
Cystic fibrosis   21
Cystoscopy   132

Dehydration   22, 65, 74
Delusions   79
Depression   11, 13
Diabetes   10, 28, 73, 85
Diabetic mononeuropathy   29
Diabetic peripheral neuropathy   29
Diabetic retinopathy   28, 85
Diagnosis   113, 114
Diarrhoea   9, 12
Differential blood count   157
Digoxin   178
  toxicity   34
Diplopia   27, 86, 87
Disability   118–123
  analysis of   122
  assessment of   120–122
  identifying causes of   123
  setting objectives for   122
Discharge note   117
Disorientation   80
Dissecting aneurysm   36

Dizziness   11
Down's syndrome   51
Drugs   15
   in serum   190
Dupuytren's contracture   22, 65
Dysarthria   78
Dysdiadochokinesis   94
Dysgraphia   79
Dyslexia   78
Dyspareunia   10
Dysphagia   9
Dysphasia   78
Dysphonia   78
Dyspnoea   8, 33, 47

Echocardiography   141
Ectopics   8, 173
Efficiency   186
Effusions
   joint   30
   pleural   58, 60, 61
Ejection click   42
Elderly
   care of the   118–123
   communication in the   122
Electrocardiogram (ECG)   159
   looking at   183
   24-hour tape recording   143
Electroencephalogram   154
Emphysema   58
Empyema   21, 55
Endocrine diseases   28–9
Endoscopic retrograde
      cholangio-pancreatography   150
Endoscopy   123, 150
Eosinophils   62
Epididymes   73
Epilepsy   11
Erythema, palms   21
Erythrocyte sedimentation rate
      (ESR)   188
Euthyroid   27
Examination, basic   108
Exercise test   140
Exophthalmos   27
External jugular vein   36
Extrapyramidal dysfunction   94, 107
Extrasystoles   34
Eyes   23

Facial nerve   89
Faints   11
Fallot's tetralogy   22
Family history   14
Fasciculation   92

Fatigue   7
Felty's syndrome   31
Fever   7
Fibrosing alveolitis   21, 55
Fibrosis, lung   56
Fine needle aspiration   133
Fits   11
Flexible bronchoscopy   150, 151
Foetor   23
   hepaticus   65
Foot drop   104
Function tests
   cardiovascular system   48
   lung   62
Functional disability, assessment   12
Functional enquiry   7–13
Fundi   84

Gait   11, 29, 103
Gall bladder, palpable   75
Gallop rhythm   42
Gallstones   152
Gastrointestinal investigations   150
Gastrointestinal system, history   9–10
Gastroscopy   131
Genitals, examination   73
Genito-urinary system, history   10
Glaucoma   84
Glomerular filtration rate   154
Glossopharyngeal nerve   90
Gout   12, 22, 31
Graham–Steell murmur   50
Gram stain, urine   153
Grand mal epilepsy   12
Guarding   68
Gums   23
Gynaecomastia   65

Haematological investigations   156
Haematology, normal values   187
Haemoptysis   8
Haemorrhoids   9
Hair   12, 27
Hallucinations   79
Handicap   118
Hands   20
Headache   10
Hearing   10
Heart attacks   14
Heart block
   complete   182
   first-degree   180
   second-degree   181
Heart sounds
   I   41

II 41
III 42
IV 42
  paradox 42, 44
  splitting 42
Heat intolerance 12
Heberden's nodes 31
Hemiplegia 92, 95
Hepatic encephalopathy 74
Hepatitis, serum 10
Hepatojugular reflex 37
Herniae
  direct 72
  femoral 72
  indirect 72
High blood pressure 13
Higher cerebral functions 77
Hip 98
History
  past 13–14
  taking 4–17
Hobbies 15
Holmes–Adie pupil 86
Homonymous hemianopia 83
Horner's syndrome 85
Hydrocoele 73
Hydrogen
  breath test 152
  MRI 139
Hydronephrosis 70
Hypercalcaemia 23
Hypercapnia 55
Hypercholesterolaemia 33
Hyperglycaemia 158
Hyperlipidaemia 23, 33
Hypertension 72
  grading 84
Hypertensive retinopathy 84
Hyperthyroidism 13
Hypertonia 94
Hypertriglyceridaemia 33
Hypoglossal nerve 92
Hypoglycaemia 158
Hypopituitary 28
Hypothyroidism 13, 28
Hypotonia 94
Hypotonic posture 93
Hypoxia 55
Hysterical gait 104

Icterus 23, 65
Illusions 79
Impairment 118
  assessment of 119–120
Incidence 186

Incontinence 123
Indigestion 9
Infarction, myocardial 161
Infectious endocarditis 21, 33, 51
Inflammatory bowel disease 9
Injection 9
Inspection 19
Instrumental activities of daily living
  (IADL) 121
Intercourse 10
Intermittent claudication 72
Internal jugular vein 37
Interpretation of results 186
Intestinal obstruction 74
Intravenous pyelogram 154
Investigations, interpretation 185
Iron deficiency anaemia 21, 65
Irritability 12
Ischaemic heart disease 7, 161, 167

Jaundice 9, 13, 23, 75
  obstructive 10, 75
Jaw
  jerk 89
  muscles 88
Joints 12, 22, 29
  interphalangeal 12, 31
  metacarpophalangeal 12, 31
Jugular veins 36
Jugular venous pressure 36
Junctional ectopics 174

Kernig's sign 106
Ketosis 23
Kidney 13
Knee 98
  reflexes 99
Koilonychia 21, 65
Kyphosis 29

Laboratory results, normal values 187
Laparoscopy 132
'Lead pipe' rigidity 94
Left heart failure 8, 47
Left ventricular aneurysm 40
Left ventricular hypertrophy 40, 166
Legs 97
  basic examination 109
Leischman's stain 157
Leuconychia 21, 65
Leukaemia 26
Lid lag 28
Light reflex 85
Light touch 102
Limbs and trunk 92

Liver   68
  disease, chronic   65
  failure   65
  flap   65
  metastases   69
Locomotor system   29
  history   12
Loin pain   10
Lordosis   29
Lower motor neurone lesion   89, 106
Lumbar puncture   155
Lumps   7, 25
Lung abscess   21, 55, 58
Lymph nodes   23, 25, 67
Lymphoma   25, 69

M mode echocardiography   141
Magnetic resonance imaging (MRI)   138
Malignant hypertension   11
Manubriosternal angle   37
Marfan's syndrome   51
Masses, palpation   70
Melaena   9
Memory   80
Menace reflex   83
Meningeal irritation   106
Meningitis   150
Menstruation   10
Mental disease   14
Mental test score   120
Mesothelioma   55
Metabolic acidosis   146
Metabolic alkalosis   147
Metal prosthetic valves   51
Mitral incompetence   43, 44, 45, 49
Mitral stenosis   9, 40, 43, 45, 49
Monilia   66
Monoplegia   95
Mood   77
Mouth   22
Murmurs   44, 45
  early systolic   45
  mid systolic   45
  pan systolic   45
Muscle
  power   94
  wasting   92
  weakness   29
Myasthenia   95
Myelofibrosis   69
Myocardial infarction   8, 161, 167
Myocardial ischaemia   167

Nails   21
Nausea   9

Neck stiffness   81
Necrobiosis lipoidica   28
Needle biopsy   133
Nervous system
  examination   76
  history   10–11
Neurological investigations   154
Nipples   26
Nocturia   10
Notes   111
Nuclear magnetic resonance (NMR)   138
Numbness   11
Nystagmus   87
  cerebellar   87
  vestibular   87

Obesity   28
Obsessions   79
Obstructive airways disease   22, 56, 63
Oculomotor nerve   86
Oedema
  ankle   48
  pitting   48
  sacral   48
Olfactory nerve   81
Opening snap   43
Operation notes   116
Ophthalmic nerve   85
Optic atrophy   84
Optic chiasma   83
Optic nerve   82, 83
Orchitis   73
Orientation   80
Orthopnoea   8, 33
Osler's nodes   21
Osteoarthritis   12, 22, 30, 32

P mitrale   163
P pulmonale   163
P wave   163
Pain   102
Palmar erythema   21, 65
Palpation   19
Palpitations   8, 12
Papilloedema   27, 84
Paralytic ileus   71
Paralytic strabismus   87
Paraplegia   95
Parietal lobe lesion   79
Parkinson's disease   92, 103, 107
Paroxysmal nocturnal dyspnoea   8
Paroxysmal tachycardia   8
Patent ductus arteriosus   51
Patients   128

Peak flow 147
  meter 63
Peau d'orange 26
Pectus excavatum 56
Per rectum examination 73
Per vagina examination 73
Percussion 18, 57
Perfusion scan 148
Pericardial rub 46, 51
Peritonitis 75
Perseveration 79
Personal history 14–16
Perthe's test 54
Petechiae 20
Phosphorus MRI 139
Pink puffer 64
Pins and needles 11
Plantar reflexes 100
Pleural rub 60
Pleuritic pain 7
Pneumothorax 58, 61
Podagra 31
Polyarthritis 30
Polycystic kidneys 70
Polyuria 10
Portal hypertension 74
Position sense 101
Post-operative notes 116
Postural hypertension 74
Praecordium 39
Pregnancy 27
Presentations to doctors 124
  brief follow-up 127
  new case on ward round 127
Prevalence 186
Problem list 113
Proctoscopy 132
Progress notes 115
Proliferative retinopathy 85
Proprioception 101
Proptosis 27
Prostatism 10
Psoriasis 32
Ptosis 87
Pulmonary area 41
Pulmonary embolism 9
Pulmonary hypertension 38
Pulmonary osteopathy 30
Pulmonary stenosis 38
Pulses 53
  brachial 52
  carotid 52
  dorsalis pedis 52
  femoral 52
  jugular venous 36

  popliteal 52
  posterior tibial 52
  radial 34, 52
Pulsus paradoxus 34
Pupils 85
Pus cells 62
Pyelonephritis 10
Pyloric stenosis 9, 75

QRS axis 170
QRS complex 164
Q wave, pathological 166

Radiology 133
Radionucleotide studies 137
Râles 60
Rash 7, 20
Reasoning 81
Rebound tenderness 68
Rectal examination 73
Re-entry, tachycardias 175
Reinforcement 99
Renal artery stenosis 72
Renal investigations 152
Respiratory acidosis 146
Respiratory alkalosis 146
Respiratory investigations 145
Respiratory system
  basic examination 108
  history 7–9
Reticuloses 25
Rheumatic fever 14, 51
Rheumatoid arthritis 12, 22, 31
Rheumatoid nodules 31
Right heart failure 8, 37, 48
Right ventricular heave 39
Right ventricular hypertrophy 40, 166
Rigid bronchoscopy 150, 151
Rigidity 68
Rinne's test 90
Romberg's test 105
Ronchi 60

Sciatica 106
Sclera 23
Scoliosis 29
Scotomata 83
Sensation 101
Sensitivity 185
Sensory ataxia 104
Sensory inattention 83, 102
Serial investigations 116
Sex 10
Shuffling gait 104
Sigmoidoscopy 132

Sinus arrhythmia   34
Sinus bradycardia   180
Skin
  testing for allergens   148
  tethering   27
Skull   81
Sleep   11
Smoking   9, 15
Snellen's card and test type   82
Social history   14–16
Spasm   92
Spastic gait   103
Specificity   85
Speech   78
Sphincter disturbance   11
Sphygmomanometer   35
Spider naevi   65
Spine   29, 81
Spirometry   147
Spleen   69
  enlarged   75
Splinter haemorrhages   21
Sputum   8, 62
Squint   87
ST segment
  depression   169, 170
  raised   167, 168
Staining method   153
Starvation   23
Status asthmaticus   34
Steatorrhoea   9
Stereognosis   102
Sternomastoid   55
Straight leg raising   106
Strap muscles   55
Striae   28
Stridor   55
Subarachnoid haemorrhage   156
Supraventricular tachycardia   178
Swallowing   9
Sweats, night   7
Sydenham's chorea   51
Syncope   9

T wave
  inversion   169, 170
  tall   169, 170
Tabes dorsalis   105
Tachycardia   175
Tamponade   34, 37
Taste   89
Technetium-99, 138
Teeth   23
Telangiectasia   65
Tendon reflexes   96

  arms   96
  legs   99
Tendons   33
  Achilles   33
Testes   73
Tetraplegia   95
Thermal sensation   102
Thrills   40
Throat   23
Thyroid   26
  cyst   27
  disease   12, 27
Thyroiditis, autoimmune   27
Thyrotoxicosis   27, 35, 51, 92
Tone   94
Tongue   22
Tonsils   23
Tophi   12, 31
Torsion of testes   73
Toxic levels   186
Trachea   55
Transfusion   9
Transillumination   25
Trapezius muscle   91
Travel   9, 15
Tremor   27
  Parkinson's   92
  thyrotoxicosis   92
Trendelenburg's test   53
Tricuspid area   40
Tricuspid incompetence   38
Tricuspid stenosis   38
Trigeminal nerve   88
  mandibular branch   88
  maxillary branch   88
  ophthalmic branch   88
Trochlear nerve   86
Trunk   97
Tuberculosis   9, 13
Turner's syndrome   51
Two-point discrimination   102
Two-dimensional echocardiography   141

Ultrasound   130
Upper motor neurone lesion   89,
    100, 106
Urine   10
  microscopy   153
  testing   152
  24-hour normal values   190

'v' wave of JVP   38
Vaginal bleeding   10
Vaginal discharge   10
Vaginal examination   73

Vagus nerve   91
Valgus deformity   30
Varicose veins   53
Varus deformity   30
Vein, saphenous   53
Venography   136
Ventilation scan   148
Ventricular ectopics   174
Ventricular septal defect   50
Ventricular tachycardia   179
Ventriculography   143
Vertigo   11
Vibration sense   101
Virchow's node   24, 65
Vision   10
Visual acuity   82
Visual fields   82
Vitalograph   148
Vocal resonance   60
Voice   12

Vomiting   9
VQ scan   148, 149

Water hammer pulse   50
Weakness   11
Weber's test   90
Weight   7, 12
Wenkebach heart block   34, 181
Wheezing   55, 60
Whispering pectoriloquy 60
Wolff–Parkinson–White syndrome   176
Worries   11
Wrist drop   92

Xanthelesma   33
Xanthochroma   155
Xanthomata   33

'y' descent of JVP   38